SUPERBUGS

SUPERBUGS

How to prevent the next global
health threat

Victoria Turk

Cornerstone Press

1 3 5 7 9 10 8 6 4 2

Cornerstone Press
20 Vauxhall Bridge Road
London SW1V 2SA

Cornerstone Press is part of the Penguin Random House group of companies whose addresses can be found at global.penguinrandomhouse.com.

Penguin
Random House
UK

First published in the UK by Cornerstone Press in 2022

www.penguin.co.uk

A CIP catalogue record for this book is available from the British Library.

ISBN 9781847943316

Typeset in 9.5/18 pt Exchange Text
by Integra Software Services Pvt. Ltd, Pondicherry

Printed and bound in Great Britain by Clays Ltd, Elcograf S.p.A.

The authorised representative in the EEA is Penguin Random House Ireland, Morrison Chambers, 32 Nassau Street, Dublin D02 YH68.

Penguin Random House is committed to a sustainable future for our business, our readers and our planet. This book is made from Forest Stewardship Council® certified paper.

MIX
Paper from
responsible sources
FSC® C018179
FSC
www.fsc.org

Contents

Introduction: The post-antimicrobial world

When the novel coronavirus SARS-CoV-2 started spreading around the world in late 2019 and early 2020, infecting people with Covid-19, we were caught off-guard. It was a new virus: we didn't know of any drugs that could cure the disease and we had no vaccines to protect against it. Hospitals were overwhelmed with infected patients, and doctors were limited in what they could do to help. The virus spread quickly, causing a global pandemic. The only way to stem the flow was to slow transmission by keeping people away from one another. Families and friends were separated, businesses shut, borders across the globe closed. By early 2022, more than six million people had died of the virus,[1] with many more deaths likely caused by indirect effects of the pandemic, such as disruption to health services.

Covid-19 was something we hadn't seen before and we had no medicines to defend ourselves against it. But it's not only new pathogens, like SARS-CoV-2, that pose a threat to global human health. Antimicrobial resistance means that existing bugs – ones we perhaps don't worry too much about – are becoming resistant to the treatments we have come to take for granted, such as antibiotics. As this resistance becomes more common, we could find ourselves in a similar situation: facing infectious diseases with limited treatment options. Our experience under Covid-19 may have given us a glimpse of that future. 'It shows what the world would be like if we had resistance to all known antibiotics,' says Jessica Boname, former head of antimicrobial resistance at the UK's Medical Research Council. 'We would be in the Covid-19 world.'

Antimicrobial resistance (AMR) occurs when microbes develop resistance to antimicrobial drugs. Today, if we get an infection, we generally expect that we can go to the doctor and get some medicine to treat it. But if the microbes causing the infection are resistant to that medicine, the infection may not go away. We might go on to try another drug, and another, and another, but if the microbes are resistant to those too, we're back at square one. Microbes that are able to resist multiple antimicrobials are sometimes referred to as 'superbugs' – and they can be very difficult to treat.

You might have heard of antibiotic resistance, which refers specifically to bacteria becoming resistant to antibiotics. Antimicrobial resistance is a broader term that covers bacteria but also other microbes such as fungi, parasites and viruses, which can develop resistance to antifungal, antiparasitic and antiviral drugs. Bacterial infections are often the focus of discussions on antimicrobial resistance, as these are where we most rely on antimicrobials, and where resistance therefore poses a particularly grave threat. But drug resistance in other pathogens is also a growing issue.

The stakes are high. If antimicrobial resistance is left to rise unchecked, we may no longer be able to knock out common infections with a simple prescription. Illnesses caused by resistant pathogens will require longer, more costly treatment. In more and more cases, we may not be able to treat a resistant infection at all.

And it's not just routine infections that will become more dangerous as we lose more antimicrobials from our medical arsenal. Much of modern medicine is built on the assumption that we can easily fight or prevent infection. If this is no longer the case, these foundations start to crumble. Take surgery: antibiotics are given as a preventative measure before and after many operations that have a high risk of infection, such as hip replacements, organ transplants or Caesarean sections. If we can no longer count on antimicrobials being effective, surgery will become much more risky. In some cases, it may be unviable: the risk of getting an untreatable infection will simply be too high. Cancer treatment is also heavily reliant on antimicrobials. Chemotherapy weakens the immune system, making it much more likely for those undergoing treatment to get infections. If our antimicrobials aren't reliable, chemotherapy becomes more hazardous. Patients could find themselves having to balance the risk posed by their progressing cancer with that of catching a resistant infection. The treatment could become nearly as dangerous as the disease.

We imagine that, with all our scientific and technological advances, medicine can only move forward, but antimicrobial resistance raises the prospect of it plummeting backwards instead. In an extreme scenario, we could enter a post-antimicrobial era, which (aside from some advances in hygiene practices) could look a lot like pre-antimicrobial times. Danilo Lo Fo Wong, regional adviser for the control of antimicrobial resistance at the World Health Organization's (WHO) Europe office, says that, if antimicrobial resistance is allowed to increase to this extent, then 'basically the last 70, 80 years of modern medicine will get lost, and we'll go back to the era before penicillin was discovered'.

What's more, Boname says, the impact could go beyond human health. Covid-19 only really impacted people, 'whereas if certain bacteria become completely resistant to treatment, they may well be pathogens which infect animals as well as humans, and we're in real trouble because we start wiping out animal populations as a food source'.

But antimicrobial resistance isn't a hypothetical doomsday scenario or a concern for the future; for many, it's already here. Millions of people experience an antimicrobial-resistant infection every year. Some don't recover. One recent study estimated that as many as 1.3 million people died directly of bacterial antimicrobial resistance in 2019 – that's more people than die of HIV or malaria.[2] The death rate was highest in West Africa, but no country is immune. The US Centers for Disease Control and Prevention (CDC) reports that more than 2.8 million resistant infections occur in the country every year, with more than 35,000 people dying as a result[3] – around the same number as die in road traffic accidents.[4]

The problem is getting worse. The WHO puts antimicrobial resistance in its top ten threats to global health, right up there with climate change and a global influenza pandemic, and says that 'antibiotic resistance is rising to dangerously high levels in all parts of the world'.[5] The growing threat of antimicrobial resistance has been called a 'silent pandemic' and a 'slow tsunami'. Lo Fo Wong compares it to the flow of molten lava – not a sudden eruption, like the Covid-19 pandemic, but a steady creep that can be deadly where it lands. 'It's here,' he says. 'And it's only going in one direction, unless we do something about it.'

1
Resistance rising

It was just a UTI. Helen Osment, a fundraiser from Hertfordshire, UK, had had urinary tract infections before, and she knew the symptoms. When she called the doctor with pain, a burning sensation and blood in her urine, they prescribed a course of antibiotics – a few days of nitrofurantoin. That should take care of it. But this time, her UTI didn't go away. It got worse. The pain was bad and she started feeling feverish and wasn't able to go to work. As her symptoms failed to improve, she felt uncomfortable and miserable. 'I think it can affect you mentally when you have one, it can make you feel quite sort of down and low,' she says.

Her doctor tried another antibiotic, trimethoprim, but the infection remained. Still feeling awful, she asked the doctor for 'something stronger', keen to feel better and get back to work. Options were limited by the fact that Osment had been deemed allergic to penicillin as a child, and this was flagged on her records. She was prescribed ciprofloxacin but reacted badly: she felt heart palpitations and pain in her knee, which turned out to be tendinitis, a potential side-effect of the drug. She visited a walk-in centre, where she was told to stop taking it and was put on a longer course of nitrofurantoin. Eventually, after weeks, the infection went away, although it took a while for Osment to fully recover.

It's a common story, and one that will only become more so as antimicrobial resistance increases. A simple infection – one that usually wouldn't raise an eyebrow – becomes a bigger problem, as the drugs we assume will be readily effective suddenly aren't.

For Osment, it was the first of several encounters with antimicrobial resistance. Later, when she was pregnant, she found out she was carrying Group B streptococcus, a common bacterium that is usually harmless to adults but can pose a risk to newborn babies. She was given antibiotics during labour, but due to resistance, on top of her penicillin allergy, the choice was limited. The experience caused her anxiety. 'It was quite a strong antibiotic that they had to offer, so I was worried about weighing up the risks and benefits,' she says. Resistance struck again when her baby was six weeks old and she developed mastitis, an infection of breast tissue most common in breastfeeding women. Reluctant to take antibiotics again, she tried to resolve it herself, but as it got worse she was prescribed a course of erythromycin. Her condition deteriorated. Feverish and in so much pain she couldn't even pick up her baby, she ended up in A&E. 'I was thinking, oh surely they'll just give me some more antibiotics,' she says. 'I didn't realise how ill I was.'

The mastitis had formed a large abscess, and Osment had developed sepsis – a life-threatening condition caused by the body's response to an infection. Luckily, this was caught early, and after being hospitalised and put on a different antibiotic intravenously, she beat the infection and recovered.

Osment's experiences had a lasting impact. She was anxious about getting ill again. 'It definitely massively affected my mental health,' she says. Before she experienced a resistant infection herself, she had been aware that antimicrobial resistance was an issue, but she had never expected to be directly affected. 'It just goes to show that it can happen to anybody, and things can escalate very quickly,' she says. She now shares her story through the charity Antibiotic Research UK, to help raise awareness of antimicrobial resistance. (She has also since found out that she is not actually allergic to penicillin, or perhaps has outgrown her allergy; while about 10 per cent of people in the UK and US report having a penicillin allergy – often diagnosed after having a rash as a child – it's estimated that only around 10 to 20 per cent of these are truly allergic.)[1]

Osment's experience is far from unusual, and in many respects she is lucky. It's hard to know exactly how many people are affected by antimicrobial resistance, and how many end up dying of resistant infections. Some countries have better surveillance and reporting systems than others, and it may not always be possible to tell if antimicrobial resistance has caused someone's death. After all, antimicrobial resistance is not a disease in itself, but a complication of many possible illnesses.

If it's hard to estimate the current burden of AMR, it's even harder to predict what it could be in the future. One influential report led by British economist Jim O'Neill in 2014 suggests that, in a worst-case scenario, 10 million deaths could be attributable to AMR every year by 2050 – more than are currently caused by cancer.[2] It may be unlikely we'll ever see that kind of number, but the message is clear: left unchecked, resistance will only get worse.

So, how did we get here?

The ideal substance

The discovery of the first antibiotic happened by chance. In August 1928, Alexander Fleming, a Scottish researcher working at St Mary's Hospital in London, went on holiday. On leaving his laboratory, he abandoned some Petri dishes in which he had been growing cultures of *Staphylococcus aureus*, a bacterium that can cause everything from pimples to meningitis.

When he returned in September, he observed something quite odd. One of the dishes was contaminated with a fungal mould, blue-green in colour.[3,4] Around the mould, the bacteria had become transparent and was disintegrating, yet further away from the mould it still thrived. Could it be that the mould was preventing the bacteria from growing, or even killing it?

To experiment, Fleming grew more of the mould on another dish and streaked different bacteria across it. He confirmed that the mould could kill *S. aureus*, as well as other types of harmful bacteria (although not all). And, crucially, it was not toxic to humans. He named his mould substance penicillin, after the genus of the fungus species, *Penicillium notatum*.

Initially, the full impact of Fleming's discovery was not apparent. Penicillin was seen more as a tool for researchers than a useful treatment for patients. Fleming figured that he could use it to help isolate microbes that weren't susceptible to penicillin; the penicillin would prevent any microbes sensitive to it from growing and leave the others to thrive. 'Had I been an active clinician I would doubtless have used it more extensively than I did therapeutically,' he said in his Nobel Lecture in 1945, when he was awarded the Nobel Prize in Physiology or Medicine for his work. 'As it was, when I had some active penicillin I had great difficulty in finding a suitable patient for its trial, and owing to its instability there was generally no supply of penicillin if a suitable case turned up.'[5]

But other researchers – most notably Ernst Chain and Howard Florey, who shared the Nobel Prize with Fleming – were able to purify penicillin and turn it into a pharmaceutical that could be mass-produced. Today, it's hard to overstate the impact of Fleming's discovery on the history of medicine. Here was a drug that could kill bacteria responsible for some of our most common ailments. We still use various different kinds of penicillin antibiotics to treat bacterial infections of the ear, throat and skin, as well as pneumonia, anthrax, diphtheria, syphilis and more. Fleming's breakthrough opened the floodgates to the discovery of all kinds of antibiotics to target different harmful bacteria, as well as other antimicrobials to fight infections caused by different types of pathogens.

Reflecting in his 1945 lecture on a visit he had made to large penicillin factories in the US, Fleming said that it was 'of especial interest' to him to see how his simple observation had developed into such a large industry, and 'how what everyone at one time thought was merely one of my toys had by purification become the nearest approach to the ideal substance for curing many of our common infections'.[6]

An ideal substance it was; in some ways *too* ideal, because while antibiotics were able to treat infections, some of which would otherwise be fatal, they came with a catch. The more bacteria are exposed to antibiotics, the more pressure they face to become resistant to those antibiotics – meaning that greater antibiotic use leads to greater resistance. And suddenly they were being used everywhere.

The bacterial arms race

To understand how bacteria become resistant to antibiotics, you need to know a little bit about how they work. Bacteria aren't bad; in fact, we need them to survive. There are trillions of microbes living on and in our bodies, many of them doing useful things like helping us to digest food and keeping us healthy by fending off other microbes that could cause us harm. In fact, there are around as many bacterial cells in and on you right now as there are human cells.[7] But problems arise when the wrong bacteria get in the wrong place in the wrong quantity; the balance is upset, and they can cause an infection. When this happens, if our own immune system can't set things right, we can take antibiotics in an attempt to kill or subdue the offending bacteria. But if the bacteria are resistant to the antibiotic, the drug will not have the intended effect and they can continue to wreak havoc, causing further illness.

Most antibiotics aren't so much created as discovered. They exist in nature: in the soil, up your nose, inside your gut. They are substances produced by bacteria – or, as in the case of penicillin, fungi – to fend off other kinds of bacteria that are competing for resources. It's a constant battle on a micro scale: different microbes squabbling over nutrients, producing antibiotics that target their rivals to keep them at bay. Some antibiotics are broad-spectrum, meaning they work against a large range of different bacteria, while others are narrow-spectrum, only targeting particular types.

We tend to imagine bacterial cells as empty bags of liquid, says Mark Webber, a group leader specialising in the evolution of antimicrobial resistance at the Quadram Institute in Norwich, UK. But this isn't the case. 'If you look at what's in a cell, it's full of stuff, and all of the things inside the cell are doing things,' he explains. 'So it's like a kind of little city full of nano machines, building stuff.' They're working away, copying DNA, building proteins, and doing all the other things a bacterial cell needs to do to survive and thrive.

Antibiotics work by disrupting some of this critical machinery, binding to it and stopping it from functioning – 'kind of like sticking a spanner in an engine,' Webber says. Antibiotics usually target one of the bacterial cell's core functions, such as its ability to synthesise its cell wall, replicate DNA or produce proteins. An antibiotic can either kill bacteria (known as a 'bactericidal' antibiotic) or inhibit their growth (a 'bacteriostatic' antibiotic).

Take penicillin as an example. Nowadays, we have several different penicillin-type antibiotics; you might be prescribed amoxicillin for a chest infection or flucloxacillin for mastitis.[8] Penicillins belong to a large and commonly used group of antibiotics known as the beta-lactam antibiotics, which work by preventing certain bacteria from building their cell walls. The penicillin binds to a protein that is needed to build part of the cell wall, inhibiting it from doing its job and killing the cell in the process. Because human and bacterial cells work differently, antibiotics don't have the same deadly effect on our own cells.

But bacteria don't just give up and die out. Just as bacteria are able to produce their own antibiotics, so they can come up with ways to resist them. Bacteria that were previously susceptible to antibiotics can develop resistance in two main ways. The first is by mutation. Every time a bacterial cell divides and multiplies (which is often – *Escherichia coli* can double every 20 minutes in ideal laboratory conditions),[9] its DNA has a chance to randomly mutate in a way that gives the resulting bacteria a new property. This is happening constantly in the background, and often it's nothing we need to worry about. 'The interesting thing about bacteria is they grow to very large populations and they reproduce very quickly, so they have an awful lot of generations,' Webber says. 'And every time a bacteria grows, it can potentially introduce a mutation within its genome somewhere.' The problem occurs when one of these mutations makes the bacteria resistant to an antibiotic.

A mutation may cause a change in the bacterial cell wall or cell membrane that prevents the antibiotic from getting into the cell in the first place.[10] Or it could give the bacteria the ability to actively pump the antibiotic out using something called an efflux pump. Other mechanisms of resistance can directly destroy the antibiotic by producing enzymes that inactivate the drug. Some bacteria, for example, can produce enzymes called beta-lactamases, which break down a crucial component of beta-lactam antibiotics such as penicillin. Mutations can also shield the target of the antibiotic so that the drug can't get to where it needs to go in the cell, or modify it so that the antibiotic doesn't have the same effect. Alternatively, the cell can develop a different way to complete a critical task – build a different piece of machinery – so that it can keep functioning even if the antibiotic takes out its intended target.

Different bacteria may be more likely to develop some of these mutations over others, but the toughest to treat – the superbugs – can have several resistance mechanisms in play at once.

The second way that bacteria can gain resistance is through a process called horizontal gene transfer. This is when one bacterial cell passes its resistance genes to another, which can happen via a few different methods. Some bacteria can pick up DNA from the environment around them. Viruses that infect bacteria, called bacteriophages (more on these in Chapter 5), can also carry bacterial DNA from cell to cell. And some bacteria can pass resistance genes to neighbouring cells via DNA molecules called plasmids. 'That's important, because you can get plasmids with lots of different resistance genes on them,' Webber says. 'A bacteria can be completely susceptible to all the antibiotics that we might want to use to treat it, and if it gets given a plasmid that has five resistance genes, it can be resistant to all five of those antibiotics in one go.'

All of this can happen naturally, without any human intervention. Bacteria that have resistance genes to the antibiotics we use today have been found in places that have never seen a manufactured pharmaceutical: in 30,000-year-old permafrost,[11] in the guts of an isolated Amazonian tribe,[12] and in caves in New Mexico that lay unexplored for 4 million years (see Chapter 3).[13]

But it's our use of antibiotics that is driving the alarming rates of antimicrobial resistance we see today – and that needs to change if we want our antimicrobials to remain effective in the future.

Too much of a good thing

The way antimicrobial use drives resistance is quite simple. When you expose bacteria to an antibiotic, the antibiotic does its job and kills off the bacteria that are sensitive to it. But if there are any bacteria that aren't sensitive to it – that have some sort of resistance mechanism – then they survive. These bacteria can then continue to grow and reproduce to make more bacteria with that resistance mechanism. Eventually, the majority of the bacteria may be resistant.

'The potential for bugs to become resistant has always been there,' says Webber. 'But our discovery and use of antibiotics has then provided an enormous selective pressure.' A selective pressure is an external factor (in this case antibiotic exposure) that causes a certain population of an organism (in this case the drug-resistant bacteria) to more effectively survive and reproduce than others. The antibiotic exerts selective pressure because it creates an environment where resistant bacteria thrive but non-resistant bacteria struggle to survive.

Essentially, the more we use antimicrobials, the more we create the conditions for resistant microbes to evolve and multiply. And as a result, the more we use antimicrobials, the less effective they may become.

Say you have an infection – a UTI caused by *E. coli* bacteria – and you take an antibiotic, like trimethoprim, to treat it. But a minority of the bacteria causing the infection have resistance to trimethoprim. Your infection may seem to clear up initially, as all the *E. coli* that are susceptible to trimethoprim are killed, but those with resistance remain, and then they multiply. The infection is still there, and now trimethoprim has no effect; the majority of the bacteria have resistance. So you need to turn to a second antibiotic option, like nitrofurantoin, and hope that the bacteria don't have resistance to that too.

This is not an academic scenario. In England and the US, around one-third of UTIs have been found to have resistance to trimethoprim.[14, 15] Trimethoprim used to be the first-choice treatment for UTIs in England, but the National Institute for Health and Care Excellence (NICE) now only recommends prescribing trimethoprim as a first option to treat a UTI if there is a low risk of resistance. It's likely that our use – and misuse – of trimethoprim and drugs like it may have helped to drive this resistance, rendering it less effective when we now need it. It's just one example of a previously go-to treatment being struck a blow by antimicrobial resistance.

Every time we use antimicrobials, we risk driving resistance. Often, we don't have a choice: if someone has a harmful infection that their body cannot fend off by itself, they need treatment. But the problem is that we're not just using them when we really need to. Overuse and misuse of antimicrobials is a big part of the resistance problem. Doctors may prescribe antimicrobials without first testing if an infection is actually causing a patient's symptoms. Patients may take antibiotics when they have cold or flu symptoms – even though antibiotics have no effect on viruses. So while some resistance may be inevitable as we use antimicrobials to keep people healthy, this inappropriate use is exacerbating the issue.

In this sense, antimicrobials are a victim of their own success. The discovery of the first antibiotic was such a step-change in medicine that we perhaps began to take these drugs for granted and use them too much and in the wrong ways. 'It became this miracle of medicine that was perceived to be the answer to everything, so it's been used for appropriate reasons but also for inappropriate reasons,' Lo Fo Wong says.

We need to be more judicious about when we use antibiotics and not give away our 'ideal substance' so freely. 'We have the wonderful history now of many decades that these are drugs that are pretty darn safe and effective, and it's really easy to just prescribe them and use them, just in case,' says Tim Jinks, head of Infectious Diseases Interventions at health research charity Wellcome.

One reason for overuse is that antimicrobials are cheap – a good thing for those who need them, but perhaps an incentive to prescribe and take them more readily than we should. Testing for a bacterial infection can be difficult; it is often faster, cheaper and easier (and more satisfactory to the patient) to simply prescribe a course of antibiotics and see if they work.

Another reason is that, in many countries, antimicrobials are available for people to buy over the counter from pharmacies, without the need for a prescription. This can lead to them being used inappropriately – people might take the wrong kind of antibiotic for their infection, for instance, or take them for symptoms that are not caused by a bacterial infection at all. A simple solution might seem to be to make antibiotics prescription-only everywhere, but this isn't necessarily the answer. 'Morally, that sounds absolutely right,' says Muhammad Zaman, a professor of biomedical engineering at Boston University and author of the book *Biography of Resistance*.[16] 'Until you realise that, in many parts of the world, there is nobody to prescribe those drugs.' For those without access to healthcare facilities, making antibiotics prescription-only would make them unavailable to people who really need them.

In low- and middle-income countries, counterfeit or substandard antibiotics are also an issue.[17] This can complicate the resistance story: if a patient's symptoms do not improve with an antibiotic, it may be impossible to tell whether this is down to resistance to the drug or if the drug itself was faulty. A poor-quality antibiotic could also contribute to resistance by providing too low a dose of the active ingredient, such that bacteria isn't killed but is still exposed to the selective pressure that drives resistance.[18]

We don't want to stop using antimicrobials. An untreated infection poses a more immediate danger to a patient than the more abstract issue of antimicrobial resistance. Antimicrobials have revolutionised healthcare, and they save lives. It's misuse and overuse that is the problem. And this isn't only an issue in human health.

Resistance all around

We don't only expose microbes to antimicrobials when we prescribe or take them to treat an infection. Human activity is driving resistance in other ways, too. One is residue from drug-manufacturing facilities, which, if allowed to get into the environment, can expose bacteria to large amounts of antibiotics. This can create conditions for resistant bacteria to thrive. People can also be exposed to this antibiotic waste, for example when using contaminated river water. The effect could be the same as if they had taken an antibiotic. 'They will be exposed to unnaturally high levels of antibiotics or antibiotic residue without even knowing it,' Boname says. Initially, this may have no effect, but bacterial communities living in these people's microbiomes may become resistant owing to the selective pressure exerted by exposure to the antibiotic pollution. If these bacteria then start causing an infection, it may no longer respond to those antibiotics.

Another hotspot of antimicrobial pollution is hospitals. Wastewater from healthcare facilities is naturally high in both infection-causing microbes (as lots of people in hospitals are ill with infections) and drug residue (from their treatments), making it a perfect reservoir for antimicrobial resistance. One study that looked at sewage from a hospital in Scotland found that there were more antimicrobial-resistant genes in hospital wastewater than in that from the general community, and that the levels of different types of resistance genes reflected the antimicrobials given to patients.[19] Again, if these resistant bacteria get into the environment, they can spread. Sometimes, they can even give resistance to other bacteria through horizontal gene transfer. While we can't stop using antimicrobials in hospitals – this is where they're often most urgently required – we need to be better at treating effluent, says Jinks: 'Throughout the world, there is insufficient treatment of healthcare facility waste.'

And it's not only humans that consume antimicrobials. While the discovery of these drugs signalled a new chapter in human healthcare, it also presented a new tool for the treatment of animals, and particularly livestock. After all, animals get infections too. But just as in people, the overuse and misuse of antimicrobials in animals is driving growing resistance.

This was brought to global attention back in 1969, after the UK government appointed a special committee to look into the issue. The Joint Committee on the Use of Antibiotics in Animal Husbandry and Veterinary Medicine produced a report, now often referred to simply as the 'Swann Report' after the committee's chair, Michael Swann. The report found a 'dramatic increase' in the number of bacteria from animals that showed resistance to one or more antibiotics, and noted that this resistance could spread to other bacteria.[20]

The authors wrote that the use of antibiotics in animals posed a hazard to both animals and humans. Animals could get resistant infections that don't respond to antibiotics, and humans could pick up resistant bacteria from animals, either from close contact with them or from eating animal products. In some cases, the same bacteria can cause infection in animals and humans; in others, the resistant bacteria may not pose a direct threat to human health but could pass their resistance to other, more dangerous bacteria in the human gut. 'Such a chance meeting between resistant organisms and highly dangerous (pathogenic) ones could give rise to a potentially explosive situation,' wrote Swann and his committee.

The problem that the Swann Report identified was not so much about giving animals antibiotics if they had an infection. Farmers weren't only using antibiotics when livestock got sick; they used them preventatively, to try to stop animals falling ill in the first place, and as a growth promoter: pigs and poultry were found to grow faster when fed small doses of antibiotics such as penicillin, making them more economical to breed. The Swann Report estimated that in 1967 around 41 per cent of all antibiotics were consumed by animals, equating to 168 tonnes. Of this, 84 tonnes were feed additives.[21]

The Swann Report recommended that antibiotics important for human health, such as penicillin, should no longer be used in animals for growth promotion and should only be accessible by prescription. The report made an impact, but it perhaps didn't go far enough. Although it was at times scathing about the preventative use of antibiotics in agriculture, it didn't explicitly make recommendations on this, and instead suggested that veterinarians should remain free to prescribe any antibiotics they saw fit.[22] It was a compromise – and a potential loophole. Farmers who couldn't access medically important antibiotics for growth promotion could perhaps persuade a vet to sign off on them, ostensibly as a preventative treatment, resulting in the same outcome.[23]

Things are starting to change. In 2006, the UK and the EU banned the use of antibiotics in animals for growth promotion; in 2017 the US did the same. In 2022, the EU went a step further, banning the use of preventative antibiotics in groups of animals. The WHO 'strongly recommends' that the use of medically important antibiotics in animals be reduced, 'including complete restriction of these antibiotics for growth promotion and disease prevention.'[24]

Just as with human healthcare, there is no desire to remove antibiotics from the veterinary medicine cabinet. If animals are ill, we want to be able to treat them – both to help the animal in question and prevent the further spread of infection. But we need to be more careful about how we deploy them.

The dawn of antimicrobials enabled a new type of intensive farming; without having to worry so much about infection control, farmers could keep animals closer together and in less-clean conditions. But this may have led to an overreliance on antimicrobials in lieu of other practices, such as better animal husbandry. 'You can use an antibiotic to cure an infection or prevent the worst aspects of an infection when you haven't done things you really should do,' says Jinks.

The curse of the 'miracle drug' strikes again.

An uneven burden

As with many public health issues, the burden of antimicrobial resistance is not evenly shouldered. Although anyone can be affected, the brunt of the crisis is borne by those who are already vulnerable. People living in densely populated communities and with poorer sanitation are at greater risk of contracting an infection, and those with less access to healthcare services are more likely to receive inadequate treatment or suffer complications. Conflict regions, such as areas of the Middle East, may have particular issues with antimicrobial resistance thanks to a lack of medical facilities.[25] In many poorer countries, access to antimicrobials in the first place remains a more immediate problem than resistance. There are also geographical differences in terms of the pathogens of most concern and levels of resistance: the biggest threat in one country may be of little import in another.

Those who are already medically vulnerable are also at greater risk. The very young and the very old are less able to fight off infections, as are people who are immunocompromised, such as those with diabetes or people undergoing cancer treatment. Some bleak examples of the burden on vulnerable people can be seen in India, where rates of antimicrobial resistance are particularly high. A 2016 study estimated that, in India, approximately 56,500 babies in neonatal care die of sepsis after contracting resistant infections every year; the true number may be much higher.[26] In some regions, cancer patients are already having to make a tough choice between undergoing chemotherapy and risking getting a superbug, or declining chemotherapy and hoping their cancer doesn't progress.[27]

As well as geographical differences, socioeconomic factors can influence antimicrobial resistance. Those who can't afford good healthcare may be at increased risk, and those from underserved or stigmatised communities may struggle to get the care they need. There may also be a gender bias, says Lo Fo Wong. Some infections, such as UTIs, impact women more, and in some cultures women may have less access to health services.

***

It's the complex nature of antimicrobial resistance that makes it so difficult to fight. It's not a single pathogen or disease; there is no 'cure'. We will never eradicate antimicrobial resistance. All we can do is work now to reduce the threat in the future. But the long-term nature of antimicrobial resistance makes it hard to build political will; significant change won't occur in a single election cycle. Lo Fo Wong compares antimicrobial resistance to climate change: a persistent and critically important issue, but one that can easily be overshadowed by more sudden, dramatic crises. 'This is why we've been talking about it for more than 20 years and have only come so far,' he says.

Reducing antimicrobial resistance means tackling many different mechanisms of resistance, in many different pathogens, in many different situations around the world. It means developing new drugs, changing the way we diagnose and treat, and adapting behaviour on a global scale. It means addressing all of the various drivers of resistance, including in humans, animals and the environment – an approach known as 'One Health'. And it means starting now.

2

Meet the superbugs

Microbes that are resistant to multiple types of antimicrobial are referred to as multidrug-resistant (MDR), extensively drug-resistant (XDR) or, in the case where they are not susceptible to any antimicrobials, pandrug-resistant (PDR).[1] Colloquially: superbugs. It's important to remember that it's the microbe that is resistant, not the person infected. Here are just a few of the microbes that are causing concern when it comes to resistance.

Tuberculosis

As a medical officer in South Africa, Dalene von Delft didn't think to worry about tuberculosis. She'd been led to believe when she was a student that young, healthy people weren't at risk; only people who were HIV positive or otherwise immunocompromised got TB. She heard stories of other students falling ill but didn't dwell on them. After all, she worked in a hospital, and seeing TB patients was part of her job. When a family member – also a doctor – got diagnosed, she began to worry more. He was a healthy man who swam and surfed. If he could get TB, maybe it wasn't so difficult? Then she developed a dry cough.

The symptoms weren't too severe – more irritating than anything. Von Delft put them down to sinusitis but went for an X-ray just in case. 'I got the biggest shock,' she says. 'I had a prominent hole in one lung.' Given her occupation, the radiologist was convinced it was TB.

Von Delft went to see a pulmonologist to confirm the diagnosis in 2010, just days before Christmas. The pulmonologist did a bronchoscopy, inserting a tube down her throat and into her lungs to get a sample, and a couple of days later she got the result. It was TB. But there was more: it was drug-resistant.

'I can just suddenly remember being super scared of infecting others,' Von Delft recalls. She'd come around to the idea that even if she had TB, she could get treatment and recover. But with drug-resistant TB, she knew it would be more difficult. 'I can remember just shutting out my husband, shutting out everyone,' she says. 'I just wanted to make sure I didn't infect anyone else.'

Still, she was relatively sanguine about the road ahead. Aside from the cough, she felt fine; she even did weight training in her room, intent on keeping up her fitness level. But after a week or so in an isolation room in hospital, the treatment – a cocktail of antimicrobials – began to take its toll, as the side-effects kicked in: dizziness, nausea, vomiting, diarrhoea. She was having to take handfuls of pills every day; at one point it was all she could do to swallow and keep them down. She'd slowly pop them into her mouth while watching TV, feeling more and more nauseous but knowing that if she threw them up, she'd have to start again, and if she didn't take them all, the bacteria causing her TB could develop further resistance.

Her hair fell out, she lost weight, and she had severe insomnia. Worst of all, she started losing her hearing.

You may think of TB as a disease of the past. In many wealthier countries, this is largely the case. But globally, TB remains one of the top causes of death and the leading cause of death from a single infectious agent (overtaken only in 2020 and 2021 by Covid-19).[2,3] The WHO's 2020 Global Tuberculosis Report estimates that, in 2019, 10 million people fell ill with TB and around 1.4 million died of the disease. Countries with the highest rates of TB include India, Indonesia, China, Pakistan, Nigeria, Bangladesh and South Africa.[4]

TB is caused by a bacterium called *Mycobacterium tuberculosis* and usually affects the lungs. It is treatable, but antimicrobial resistance is making it harder to handle. Drug-resistant TB causes 230,000 deaths per year, accounting for more than a third of all deaths attributed to antimicrobial resistance. In 2019, close to half a million people had TB that was resistant to rifampicin, one of the most powerful go-to antibiotics for TB. Of these, the majority – 78 per cent – had infections that were also resistant to isoniazid, another first-line antibiotic for TB. An infection caused by bacteria that is resistant to both of these drugs is called multidrug-resistant TB, or MDR-TB. Less than 60 per cent of people treated for MDR-TB are successfully cured.[5]

With the two most potent drugs ruled out, treating MDR-TB requires taking a course of multiple second-line antibiotics for at least nine months, and sometimes up to 20 months. These antibiotics can have severe side-effects, as Von Delft experienced. This is often the case with antimicrobials that we hold back for use only when others fail: we keep them in reserve not only to try to prevent resistance from emerging, but also because they can have serious negative effects; we don't want to give them to people if there's a better choice.

Von Delft considers herself lucky. She was granted compassionate access (when access is permitted to an experimental treatment that wouldn't usually be authorised, if patients don't have other options) to a drug called bedaquiline, new at the time, which meant she was able to stop taking the treatment that was causing her hearing loss. After a gruelling 19 months of treatment, she made a full recovery.

But her experience illustrates why it can be so hard to get on top of TB. The microbes that cause TB can be particularly persistent and take a long time to kill, even when they aren't drug-resistant (the standard length of treatment is six months). When you take into account the length and difficulty of TB treatment, it's easy to see how patients can end up not completing it. And this helps to fuel resistance.[6] That's because if a patient's treatment is interrupted, or they do not receive the proper drugs, the bacteria causing their infection may continue to grow, and resistance can emerge. Resistant TB can then spread from person to person, especially in crowded environments.

Lack of testing is another problem: if people don't know they have TB in the first place, they won't get treatment, and if people with TB are not tested to see if it is drug-resistant, they won't get the *right* treatment.

For Von Delft, her own experience was an eye opener. 'I consider myself quite a tough person – you know, medical school's tough,' she says. 'And that was definitely one of the toughest things I had to do.' Though she tried, she wasn't well enough to work while undergoing treatment. As a doctor, she had support, but she notes that plenty of people may not have enough help – financial, emotional or practical – to see through the difficult treatment regimen.

When it comes to antimicrobial resistance, Von Delft, who now works as a GP, feels that TB is often overlooked, despite it contributing to an outsized proportion of AMR-related deaths and illness. This, she says, may partly be down to racism and social inequity. 'TB mainly affects people of colour, mainly affects people in developing countries,' she says. Following her own battle with TB, she helped to set up an organisation called TB Proof, which aims to reduce the stigma that still persists around TB and advocate for better access to high-quality treatment for all.

If there's one thing that the example of TB demonstrates, it's that antimicrobial resistance is not a problem of the future. It's already here today – and it's deadly. Gwen Knight, an associate professor at the London School of Hygiene and Tropical Medicine, worries that people too often see antimicrobial resistance as a distant issue rather than one that is currently having an impact, and that we focus disproportionately on the risks posed to high-income countries than low- and middle-income countries where the burden is already greater. 'We worry about settings in which people can afford to and are able to have hip operations and things like this,' she says. 'And maybe we should be worrying about settings where they actually just can't even afford the drugs [in the first place].'

Healthcare-associated infections

Think of the term 'superbug' and you probably have a particular image in mind: patients in hospital beds, laid low by an invisible foe; closed wards; cleaners wiping down medical equipment. The irony is that, in many ways, healthcare environments offer an ideal place for antimicrobial-resistant bugs to spread. There are lots of ill people in hospitals, bringing their germs with them. There is also a high use of antimicrobial drugs, creating conditions in which resistant bugs can thrive. And there are lots of other ill people whose immune systems may be weakened, ready for infection to strike.

Bugs can spread directly from patient to patient, or else through the hospital environment or via medical procedures. Microbes that live harmlessly on our skin, for example, can cause problems if they enter other parts of the body – which can happen as a result of injuries such as cuts or burns, during surgery, or via medical equipment such as catheters or ventilators.

A healthcare-associated infection, also called a nosocomial infection, is an infection acquired in a healthcare environment – one that the patient didn't have before they came in. And as with any infection, if antimicrobial resistance is involved, it is harder to treat.

Such is the threat that one of the biggest risk factors for getting an antimicrobial-resistant infection is staying in a healthcare facility.[7]

You've probably heard of MRSA (methicillin-resistant *Staphylococcus aureus*), a type of bacteria that is resistant to certain antimicrobials and that became well known in the UK and US for causing deadly outbreaks in hospitals, particularly in the mid-2000s. Cases of hospital-acquired MRSA in these two countries have since declined, a trajectory largely attributed to improved infection-control measures such as enhanced cleaning and better reporting systems. But MRSA is far from the only bug that poses a threat. And there is one type of bacteria that is causing particular concern.

Gram-negative bacteria

Pneumonia, bloodstream infections, urinary tract infections, gonorrhoea, wound infections, respiratory infections, stomach infections, food poisoning, meningitis … name the infection, you'll probably be able to find a Gram-negative bacteria that can cause it. And this kind of bacteria is particularly worrisome when it comes to drug-resistant infections, in healthcare environments and beyond. In 2017, the WHO published its first list of antimicrobial-resistant 'priority pathogens', highlighting some of the resistant bacteria posing the greatest risk to human health. All three of the very highest-priority pathogens on the list – resistant versions of *Acinetobacter baumannii, Pseudomonas aeruginosa* and *Enterobacteriaceae* – are Gram-negative, as are six of the remaining nine.[8]

So what is 'Gram-negative'? The term refers to the outcome of a test invented by a Danish scientist called Hans Christian Gram back in the 1880s. Gram came up with a way to stain bacteria so that they could be viewed under a microscope, a method that microbiologists still use today. The Gram stain procedure is quite straightforward: a stain called crystal violet, which turns cells purple, is first applied to the bacteria sample and fixed in place using a substance such as iodine. The slide is then flooded with a decolourising agent and another stain is applied: safranin, which is red. Bacteria that look bluey-purple under the microscope after this process are classified as Gram-positive. Bacteria that look pinky-red are Gram-negative. (Some bacteria cannot be classified using the Gram stain.)[9]

What can this tell us about the bacteria? The difference between Gram-negative and Gram-positive bacteria – the reason they turn different colours – lies in their structure, and particularly their cell wall. Gram-positive bacteria have a thick cell wall, while Gram-negative bacteria have a thinner cell wall, plus an outer membrane. It's this structure that means Gram-negative bacteria don't stain like Gram-positive bacteria do. And it also means it's harder to find antibiotics that work against Gram-negative bacteria.

The structure of Gram-negative bacteria makes them intrinsically resistant to some antibiotics. Before even taking into account mutations or selective pressure, Gram-negative bacteria simply aren't sensitive to some of the antibiotics that Gram-positive bacteria are; they just shrug them off their outer membrane, which acts like a shield. 'The double membrane that Gram-negative bacteria have can make it difficult for antibiotics to penetrate into the bacterial cell where an antibiotic or drug can reach its target molecule and disrupt it,' explains Matt Mulvey, a professor at the University of Utah whose lab focuses on *Escherichia coli,* or *E. coli,* a Gram-negative pathogen common in humans. In addition to this, Gram-negative bacteria can be particularly good at acquiring resistance to antibiotics – and they can often pass this resistance on.

As a result, we're seeing a rise in resistance among many types of Gram-negative bacteria, accompanied by a lack of new antibiotics being developed to tackle them. A 2020 WHO report found that, of 60 new antibiotic agents in development, only two were active against multidrug-resistant Gram-negative bacteria.[10]

The three most critical pathogens on the WHO's list are Gram-negative bacteria that are resistant to carbapenems, a class of antibiotics usually reserved for high-risk, multidrug-resistant infections. Carbapenem is often considered a last resort – and it's usually highly effective. Where nothing else works, doctors can reach for a carbapenem, and potentially save a life. But not when the bacteria are resistant.

In August 2016, health officials in Nevada were alerted to a case of a woman who was infected with a carbapenem-resistant *Enterobacteriacea* – a family of bacteria that contains many common pathogens including *E. coli*, *Klebsiella*, *Salmonella* and *Shigella*.[11] The woman, who was in her seventies and had recently been hospitalised while on an extended trip to India, was admitted to hospital in the US after being diagnosed with systemic inflammatory response – a condition that occurs when the body's defence system essentially overreacts to a stressor such as an infection, causing body temperature to either peak or drop, a racing heart, rapid breathing and an abnormal white blood cell count.[12] This was thought to be caused by an infected seroma – a build-up of fluid that can occur after surgery – on the woman's hip.

Clinicians took a sample of bacteria from the site and found that it was *Klebsiella pneumoniae*, a bacterium that lives happily in the gut but can cause dangerous infections when it gets elsewhere, including the urinary tract, bloodstream or surgical sites. And the *Klebsiella pneumoniae* was drug-resistant – not just to a few antimicrobials but to every antimicrobial available. The woman was put in an isolated room and precautions taken to try to stop this superbug from spreading. But the bug couldn't be treated, and she died after developing septic shock.

Tests showed that the bacteria causing the woman's infection were resistant to 26 antimicrobials, including one called tigecycline, which was developed specifically in response to increasing antimicrobial resistance. The case made headlines when it was reported in 2017; it is very rare in the US that doctors are left completely empty-handed when faced with an infection. As antimicrobial resistance grows, however, this scenario will become more common.

Clostridioides difficile: tending the gut garden

To describe the main symptom of a *Clostridioides difficile* infection just as 'diarrhoea' doesn't quite communicate the severity of the disease. 'It's the worst diarrhoea that people have ever gotten in their lives,' says Sahil Khanna, a gastroenterologist at the Mayo Clinic in Minnesota who specialises in the infection. 'It's worse than getting any kind of food poisoning. It debilitates people – [they] can't go to work, can't function.'

Those with a milder version may have three to five bowel movements a day, whereas others may have 10 or 15, even 20. In severe cases, people may need surgery. The infection often spreads in hospitals and nursing homes among already vulnerable people, and it is deadly. In the US alone, there are an estimated 223,900 infections per year and 12,800 deaths.[13] The CDC lists it as an urgent threat. The European Centre for Disease Prevention and Control estimates there are more than 120,000 cases of healthcare-associated *Clostridioides difficile* annually across the EU, resulting in a conservative estimate of 3,700 deaths.[14]

Previously called *Clostridium difficile* and often shortened to just *C. diff*, *Clostridioides difficile* is a bacterium that spreads via the faecal-oral route, a common method by which many different infections are transmitted and which is exactly what it sounds like: pathogens from faecal matter end up in the mouth. This can occur, for example, if someone touches a contaminated surface and then touches their mouth, ingesting the bacteria.

C. diff isn't often resistant to antimicrobials; it's not a 'superbug' in that sense. But it is related to the antimicrobial resistance story in another way: it is often directly caused by the use (including misuse and overuse) of antibiotics.

C. diff is all around in the environment; we all get exposed to it. But usually, the bacteria in your gut – your 'good bacteria' – prevent it from causing an infection. If you have a lower number or diversity of useful bacteria in your intestine, however, *C. diff* may move in and take a hold. And one common thing that can reduce your gut bacteria diversity? Antimicrobials. When you take an antimicrobial, it usually doesn't just kill the pathogen you're hoping to get rid of but can also have an impact on other bacteria, including those that are helpful.

Khanna uses the analogy of a garden that is full of lush green grass, until one day a raccoon comes along and digs a hole. A weed takes the opportunity to grow in that space, and eventually it tries to take over, spreading across your lawn. When you take an antimicrobial drug, your gut flora may similarly develop a 'hole' as they are killed off, leaving space for an opportunistic microbe to take advantage and grow where it shouldn't.

Things get trickier when you consider the treatment for *C. diff*. 'The treatments that we use for *C. diff*, unfortunately, are antibiotics,' Khanna explains. 'Antibiotics cause *C. diff*; antibiotics are what we use to treat *C. diff*.' One common antibiotic used to treat *C. diff* is vancomycin. Khanna compares this to spraying herbicide on the weed in your once-tidy lawn. 'It kills the weed partially but kills the grass around it,' he says. 'That's what vancomycin does: kills the *C. diff* partially ... but also does collateral damage, where it kills the useful bacteria.'

This means that, once antimicrobial treatment is completed, *C. diff* can come back. One in five people who have had a *C. diff* infection will have a recurrence within eight weeks.[15] And with each recurrence, the next becomes more likely.

For patients who suffer recurrent *C. diff* that won't go away just with antimicrobials, there is another treatment option: faecal microbiota transplantation, commonly called a faecal transplant. Here, doctors take a sample of stool from someone with a healthy gut microbiome, screen it to make sure it's free of anything harmful, and then turn it into a concoction that can be administered via a colonoscopy or enema, or in pill form. The idea is that the 'good bacteria' in the stool sample can restore balance in the patient's gut, beating back the *C. diff*. In Khanna's garden analogy, it's equivalent to stealing some grass seed from your neighbour and throwing it in the spot where you're struggling to control weeds; the grass regrows so the weeds can't take over.

Ultimately, the best way to tackle *C. diff*, like antimicrobial resistance, is better antimicrobial stewardship. By only taking antimicrobials when we need them, we reduce the risk of harmful effects. Where possible, we should use narrow-spectrum antimicrobials – ones that specifically target certain types of microbe, rather than broad-spectrum drugs that kill many – and only take them in the quantity and for the duration required (it is, however, always advisable to take antimicrobials as prescribed and to finish the course). Improving hygiene controls in healthcare environments is also an important part of the puzzle, as this reduces the spread of pathogens such as *C. diff* and other hospital-associated infections in the first place. And the development of new antimicrobials – in this case, antibiotics that are more narrowly targeted and less likely to create the conditions that allow *C. diff* to thrive – could help to reduce the burden of this deadly infection.

Beyond bacteria

While bacteria are the focus when it comes to antimicrobial resistance, owing to our outsized reliance on antibiotics compared to other types of antimicrobial, they're not the only microbes we need to keep an eye on. Others, such as fungi and viruses, can also develop drug resistance.

Take fungi. You may think of fungal infections as minor afflictions, like athlete's foot or thrush. But these microbes can cause infections that are just as serious as those caused by bacteria – and treatment options are often more limited.

In May 2021, India was in the midst of a devastating second wave of Covid-19, reporting up to 400,000 new cases and 4,500 deaths every day.[16] But for some of those recovering from the virus, a new threat set in. Indian doctors reported a rise in cases of mucormycosis, a fungal infection sometimes known as 'the black fungus'. Patients who were being treated for or had recovered from Covid-19 would present with new symptoms: swelling, headaches, eye pain, black lesions on their nose or mouth. Mucormycosis can be fatal. Those who survive often need to have an eye removed to stop the infection from reaching their brain. Patients are usually given an antifungal medication called amphotericin B, but this treatment brings its own risks. It can have severe side-effects, including kidney damage, and can itself be lethal. We don't know exactly why mucormycosis targeted Covid-19 patients, but it is thought that the use of steroids to treat the virus may be a contributing factor, as these weaken the immune system. Many of those affected also had diabetes.[17]

The severity of mucormycosis shows how difficult it can be to treat infections caused by fungi. This is because fungal cells are more similar to our own than bacterial cells are. As a result, it's difficult to develop antifungal drugs that aren't also harmful to humans. 'It means there are a very limited number of metabolic targets that you can hit in fungi that don't also hit us,' says Matthew Fisher, a professor of fungal disease epidemiology at Imperial College London. 'It also means that the antifungal drugs that we do have tend to be very toxic, so you can kill a patient with an antifungal, whereas that's generally quite unlikely with antibiotics.'

Because of this, we don't actually have many antifungals to fight fungal diseases in the first place; there are only four different classes of antifungal currently available.[18] This makes resistance a particularly worrying concern: if a fungus develops resistance to just one type of drug, treatment options quickly become very limited.

Take *Aspergillus fumigatus* as an example. Like many fungi, *Aspergillus fumigatus* is an opportunist. Its spores are everywhere in the environment; we breathe them in every day. But for people whose immune systems are compromised, such as those with cystic fibrosis or who have undergone a lung transplant, it can soon cause a dangerous infection. For this reason, these patients are usually given antifungals prophylactically over a long period of time, to prevent an infection from taking hold. This long-term exposure to the drug, however, gives more chance for drug-resistance to occur – as the cells with resistance grow and reproduce while those without resistance die – at which point the antifungal may stop working.

Patients may also get infected with *Aspergillus fumigatus* that is already resistant before it enters their body. As there are so few antifungals, we tend to use the same kinds in human healthcare and in the environment. The main treatment for *Aspergillus fumigatus* is a class of antifungals called azoles. But azoles are also used in animals, on crops and even in timber coatings to prevent wood from going mouldy. 'Humanity is a power user of azoles in the environment, and the usage is spiralling upwards,' Fisher says.

When azoles are used in the environment, they kill off most *A. fumigatus* but leave the resistant fungi to survive and multiply – and potentially be breathed in by someone vulnerable. Fisher's lab is currently working on tracking down the evolution of *A. fumigatus* resistance, using genome sequencing to see where fungi with mutations that confer resistance to azoles have evolved, in order to establish how often and from where these environmentally resistant strains establish in patients' lungs.

We certainly need to consider how we use azoles and other antifungals in the environment, but the answer isn't as simple as just banning the use of azoles outside of human health. As there are so few antifungals to choose from, there aren't many alternatives, and banning their use in agriculture could mean people going hungry as crops fall to fungal disease. 'It's an absolutely classic "One Health" problem,' Fisher says. 'You're damned if you do, you're damned if you don't here – you've got to use azoles for food security, but at the same time it's breaking down our favourite class of clinical drugs.'

As we develop more antifungals, there is an argument that we should ring-fence these for use in humans only, to try to slow the emergence and spread of resistance. But as with antibiotics, developing new antifungals is a long and costly process. We are going to need to rely on our existing frontline antifungals for a long time yet.

Fungi are also increasingly a concern when it comes to healthcare-associated infections. The past decade has seen the rise of a nasty fungal infection that spreads particularly in hospital environments: *Candida auris,* a type of yeast that can cause bloodstream infections and is often resistant to multiple antifungal drugs. In 2016, Royal Brompton Hospital in London temporarily closed its intensive care unit after an outbreak of *C. auris* that gave rise to 50 cases over 16 months, nine of which resulted in a bloodstream infection.[19] Other *C. auris* outbreaks have been reported across every continent except Antarctica.[20] 'It's a pandemic, it's a fairly silent pandemic,' Fisher says.

***

The pathogens highlighted in this chapter are just a few examples of microbes that could be ever-more dangerous thanks to growing antimicrobial resistance – ones that are already, or are at risk of becoming, 'superbugs'. But new risks may emerge. While we desperately need to focus on addressing these urgent threats, we can't stop after that. Antimicrobial resistance can affect all kinds of microbes, so fixing one problem won't solve the broader issue.

We need to change the way we use all antimicrobials, keep developing new ones, improve access to healthcare, and address issues such as poor sanitation that help pathogens to spread. And we need to keep tabs on threats, so we can identify which pathogens might cause the next superbug outbreak and take targeted action against them. Only through a global, connected effort will we keep resistance in check.

3

The search for new antibiotics

Microbiologist Hazel Barton has a very specialised set of skills. An avid cave explorer since she was 14 years old, she conducts a lot of her work underground, climbing or rappelling into cave systems to sample their unique microbiology. A professor at the University of Akron, Ohio, she works out every day to meet the physical demands of the job, so she is prepared to climb, crawl and pull herself through rock structures lit only by the headlight on her helmet, her leggings and running shirt sticking to her body in up to 100 per cent humidity. For humans, the inside of a cave is not a very welcoming place: it's dry and gritty, and the only food available is what you're able to carry in your 17kg pack. The pack never gets lighter: with nowhere to dump waste, everything has to be carried back out. 'There's no hygiene other than using a baby wipe to wipe yourself down,' Barton says.

One of the caves she regularly explores, both for work and fun, is the Lechuguilla Cave, a huge cave system in New Mexico that reaches 489m deep. Entering the cave involves getting a permit, then walking 2.5km across the desert and abseiling through a pit into an entrance chamber. After more climbing and abseiling through culverts and antechambers, you reach the actual cave, which, with a length of 242km, is one of the world's longest. As the distances from the entrance to other parts of the cave system are so long, Barton usually camps underground for around eight days at a time.

One of the unusual features of Lechuguilla Cave is its remoteness. It was cut off from the surface for 4 million years before its discovery in the 1980s, and access since has been strictly limited. So when Barton first visited the cave in her capacity as a microbiologist, she didn't expect to find much. 'We kind of thought that it was going to be a simple system – that it was so nutrient-limited there were going to be very few organisms that were adapted to extreme nutrient limitation,' she says. 'But we went in, and it turned out that it was a super-diverse community.'

It transpired that the cave offered a perfect environment for many types of microbe, and Barton now makes regular trips to sample the cave's microbiology. To do this, she swabs the walls, dilutes the samples and plates them onto agar plates to return to the lab. Her team also samples the rock to understand the geology the microbes are living on, and measures temperature, humidity and pH levels to get a sense of the conditions they experience.

One of her ambitions is to find new sources of antibiotics from environments that have not previously been tapped.

A dry pipeline

For most infections, we have multiple lines of defence. If one antimicrobial doesn't work, you try another, then another, and so on until you reach those that are held back as a last resort, to be used only in extremely limited cases so as to prevent resistance from occuring. As these antimicrobials are struck down by resistance, the obvious solution would be to make new ones. But we aren't developing them fast enough. According to the WHO, lack of innovation and funding is a major concern, with most new products in development showing little extra benefit, and few targeting some of the most urgent infections, such as those caused by Gram-negative bacteria.[1]

Most of the antimicrobial substances that we commonly use today were found in the 1940s and 1950s, soon after penicillin – a 'golden era' for antibiotic discovery. But in the following decades, discoveries of new antibiotics were few and far between. The low-hanging fruit had been found, and scientists were getting frustrated at discovering the same compounds again and again.

In the latter part of the twentieth century, a new method was adopted. Rather than screening natural compounds to search for antimicrobial substances, scientists decided to try a more targeted approach. They set out to look specifically for compounds that inhibited pathways essential to the function of bacteria. If you know a bacterium needs to create a certain enzyme to thrive, for instance, then finding a compound that inhibits the production of this enzyme could give you a promising lead for a new antimicrobial drug.

Researchers screened for these targets, moving away from natural products and turning their attention to synthetic compounds in the vast chemical libraries of research groups and pharmaceutical companies.[2] It's an approach that has been successful for discovering many kinds of drugs, but it didn't really work for antimicrobials. 'They were new technologies at the time, we thought they were going to generate lots of really useful compounds,' says Mathew Upton, a professor of medical microbiology at the University of Plymouth. 'And they basically generated nothing at all.'

It's not that we didn't find anything – promising compounds were identified – but they just didn't work in actual bacteria. When they were tested, they often couldn't enter the cell, so they couldn't access the pathway they were trying to inhibit in the first place. They were effectively useless.

And so the focus turned once again to natural substances, making the most of the tiny, living antibiotic factories in the environment all around us. These days, the way many researchers find new antibiotics is not all that dissimilar to Fleming's observation of mould on a sample dish, albeit rather more deliberate.

Ancient resistance

Gerry Wright, a professor of biochemistry and biomedical studies at McMaster University, Canada, first got interested in infectious diseases during his student days in the 1980s. It was the height of the AIDS pandemic, and he saw people around his own age getting sick and dying. It was a shock: 'I thought we were in control of these things,' he says.

After first working on antifungals, he became interested in antibiotics and particularly antibiotic resistance. This led him to conduct postdoctoral research on *enterococci* bacteria that were resistant to vancomycin, a powerful 'last-resort' antibiotic that was starting to fail for some patients. After establishing his own lab, Wright sequenced the genome of a vancomycin-*producing* bacterium as part of his research. What he found surprised him. There in the sequence were the same genes he'd observed in the vancomycin-*resistant* bacteria causing so much trouble in the clinic. In other words, the same genes appeared in both the bacteria that produced vancomycin and those that were resistant to it. 'Their genetic context was the same, their orientation was the same, their mechanisms are exactly the same,' he recalls.

It made sense, really, that vancomycin-producing bacteria would need resistance genes – to protect themselves from the very substance they were making. However, when Wright and his colleagues were sequencing some other bacteria (this was in the 1990s, when genome sequencing was harder to do), they found the same sequence of resistance genes, but this time in an entirely separate organism that didn't produce the vancomycin antibiotic, and hadn't been exposed to it in the clinic.

Why would this other organism have these resistance genes? Perhaps, he thought, there was a lot more natural resistance to antibiotics out there in the environment than people realised.

The idea inspired a project. Wright sent his students out to collect soil samples around Ontario. They then isolated some of the bacteria in the samples and screened them for resistance against 21 different antibiotics on the market at the time. Wright was blown away by the results. On average, the bacteria strains were resistant to seven or eight antibiotics.[3] A couple were resistant to 15. 'If they were in the clinic, they would be the superbugs,' Wright says. The implication was that antibiotic resistance was much more pervasive in soil organisms than had been previously understood;

it wasn't just limited to healthcare environments, where antibiotic drugs were used.

There was what Wright calls some 'sniping' at the paper. Some suggested that the soil samples his lab had collected could have been contaminated by human antibiotic use; that's why the microbes had developed resistance. So Wright went further. He looked at Canadian permafrost from 30,000 years ago – when there weren't any humans in the area, never mind anyone using antibiotics. His team sampled the ancient DNA and started probing it for resistance genes. They found some. They published their findings in the journal *Nature* with the simple title 'Antibiotic resistance is ancient'.[4] Their results, the authors wrote, 'show conclusively that antibiotic resistance is a natural phenomenon that predates the modern selective pressure of clinical antibiotic use'.

It was this work that led Wright to approach Hazel Barton about her work in the Lechuguilla Cave, which had lain untouched for 4 million years. It was the perfect place for another experiment. With Barton's help, his team tested samples from the cave – microbes that had surely never seen any externally developed antimicrobials. They found a bacterium that was resistant to 26 out of 40 antibiotics tested and had five new resistance mechanisms.[5] 'That really made the point that resistance is really old,' Wright says. 'It's hardwired into the chromosomes of bacteria around the planet.'

It was further evidence that resistance genes can, and do, occur naturally in the environment, without the selective pressure of human antibiotic use. That's not to say antibiotic use isn't a major driver of resistance – it is – but it opened up the possibility that these microbes from the environment could tell us a lot more about how resistance works and give us a head start on understanding resistance mechanisms not yet observed in the lab.

Furthermore, if antibiotic resistance genes were present in the cave microbes, it followed that those microbes might also be a good source for producing antibiotics – perhaps including some we haven't seen before. After all, the resistant bacteria must be coming into contact with something in order to bother developing and retaining resistance. 'With so much antibiotic resistance, you would assume that there would be novel antibiotics down there as well,' Barton says.

How to discover an antimicrobial

The search for novel antimicrobial compounds has taken scientists to increasingly exotic places. While Barton is exploring her ancient cave systems, Upton, the University of Plymouth microbiologist, searches deep in the ocean. Working with Kerry Howell, a professor of deep-sea ecology, he studies microbes found on samples of sponges gathered from the sea, sometimes as deep as 1.5km below the surface.

The reason for searching in places so far removed from our everyday environment – even if it is quite a mission to get there – is that it increases the chance of finding a truly novel antibiotic compound, Upton explains. Often, researchers can find a substance with promising antibiotic properties, but once they've gone through the hassle of growing the microbe in the lab and purifying the compound, they find out it is the same as, or similar to, an existing antibiotic – and will therefore likely be disarmed by the same resistance mechanisms. 'If a compound is the same as something we've seen before, or very related to it, it's probably not going to be worth developing, because any resistance mechanism that is already out there will undermine it as soon as we use it in the clinic,' Upton says.

But we don't always need to look so far away from home. In fact, Upton is currently working with one compound that was found in a sample taken from the surface of human skin.

Gerry Wright, meanwhile, has built a library of extracts from about 15,000 strains of bacteria and fungi, mainly collected from soil around Canada. His lab had already collected hundreds of samples while trying to find evidence of resistance genes in the soil, but he knew that to discover new antimicrobials would likely require many more. But going out and collecting thousands of samples of dirt to process for microbes was a time-consuming and not particularly appealing prospect.

An opportunity presented itself in the form of a student whose father worked at a bank. The bank had branches all across Canada – a country the scale of a continent, with all kinds of different landscapes: urban areas, forests, deserts, mountains, permafrost. The student's father sent a note out to the bank employees, asking if they'd like to take part in a project. All they had to do was take a spoon, dig about 5cm deep into the ground, put a sample of soil into a plastic sandwich bag, and post it to Wright's lab. Hundreds of samples came in. Now, whenever a student at the lab is going camping or hiking, they're asked to bring back a soil sample.

In the lab, the soil samples are processed in order to isolate individual microbes. Wright's lab is mainly interested in actinomycetes, a family of bacteria that is a source of many antibiotics. They dry out their soil samples, add a bit of water, streak the mixture on a Petri dish of agar and see what appears. 'You get like a zoo of things growing up,' Wright says. Once they've isolated a particular bacterial strain, he and his team grow it in a Petri dish for a week or so, then grind the whole lot up – including the bacteria and whatever substances they might have produced – and extract everything they can from it. These extracts are inducted into the Wright Actinomycete Collection (WAC). 'I call it our collection of brown goos,' Wright says.

One way to test for an antimicrobial substance is much like Fleming's mould-covered Petri dish: grow one type of microbe, then grow another on top of it, and see if one inhibits the other. But other screening techniques can help to narrow down the search for compounds of interest.

Wright's lab first screen their 'brown goos' for antimicrobial activity. If they find it, they then sequence the genomes of the associated bacterial strains and use software to search for clusters of genes that we know to be associated with producing antimicrobial compounds. Find such a cluster and you might be onto something.

Wright's team also uses resistance itself to help further winnow their search to focus only on compounds that haven't been discovered before. 'We don't want to spend a lot of time isolating tetracycline again,' Wright says. They've built up a collection of genes associated with antimicrobial resistance, which they use to screen their sequenced genomes against.[6] This is because a microbe producing an antimicrobial substance needs itself to have resistance to it as a self-defence mechanism – otherwise it would cause itself harm. So, if the researchers find known resistance genes, they can rule out the compound, as it's likely something they already know about.

If, however, they find a promising gene cluster but *don't* find any known resistance genes, then they may be on track to finding a new antimicrobial substance. 'Finding new antibiotics is like looking for a needle in a haystack,' Wright says. 'So what we're always trying to do is make that haystack as small as possible, and using resistance as a filter helps make the haystack very small.'

In 2020, Wright and colleagues published a paper in *Nature* about an antibiotic they'd discovered this way that had a different mode of action.[7] 'We used the absence of [known] resistance as the strategy to go after those molecules,' he says. 'That helped us decide that that was an appropriate place to look.'

The Great Plate Count Anomaly

There's a mystery – a paradox, almost – that has plagued microbiologists for more than a century. All sorts of microbes grow in all sorts of places – except, it seems, when you try to culture them in the lab. There can be billions of bacteria in a single spoonful of soil; dilute your sample and you can observe them through a microscope. But try to grow them in a Petri dish full of agar, and you'll end up with a lot fewer. Orders of magnitude fewer. This mismatch between the number of bacteria in an environment and the number that we can actually culture is sometimes known as 'The Great Plate Count Anomaly', and it means that microbiologists have largely been working with just a tiny fraction of the bacteria out there. Yet those bacteria that we have so far been unable to culture may also produce natural antibiotic substances. Imagine what we might be able to find if we could grow more of them.

It's a riddle that Kim Lewis and Slava Epstein, both professors at Northeastern University and co-founders of NovoBiotic Pharmaceuticals, have tried to solve. The problem, Epstein explains, is that we don't know much about these so-far-uncultured microbes, precisely because we haven't been able to grow them. So as a result, we don't know what conditions would enable them *to* grow. It's a chicken-and-egg-style dilemma. 'How would you know the properties of that which by definition is unknown?' he asks. 'That's a conundrum.'

What we do know is that these microbes live happily in the environment in which they are found. We know they grow in those conditions, even if we don't know what the conditions are. So instead of taking them to a Petri dish, why not take the Petri dish to them? Epstein compares the idea to growing a plant from seed. You can plant the seed in soil, water it, and watch it germinate. Within the soil, countless interactions are happening between the seed, soil particles and microbes, but a gardener doesn't need to know what they are in order to have a successful harvest. You don't need to know *how* to grow if you know *where* to grow.

To do this for microbes, Epstein and his team came up with a device called the isolation chip, or iChip. It's a device that consists of a plate containing many small holes. Once you've got your microbes from the environment all mixed up with a gelling agent such as agar, you can dip the chip into the mixture and each hole will fill with a plug of this microbial goo. The size of the holes means that, on average, just one bacterial cell will be caught in each – successfully isolating the microbes from one another. Membranes are placed on either side of the plate, keeping the microbial cells in place but allowing chemicals to penetrate. You can then place the whole plate back into the environment where you got the sample from in the first place – in soil, on sand, or in the ocean, for instance.

Leave the plate for a while, and when you return and inspect the plugs, you may find that, although you won't know how you've done it, you have successfully cultivated microbe colonies that previously refused to be cultured. To see if any of these microbes produce an antibiotic substance, smear a bacterium such as *Staphylococcus aureus* over the plate and see if there are any holes around which it doesn't grow. *Voilà*, you may have discovered a new antibiotic substance, produced by a previously uncultured microbe.

In a 2015 article in *Nature*, Lewis, Epstein and colleagues reported finding one such antibiotic, produced by a previously undescribed bacterium that had been cultured using the iChip. They called the antibiotic teixobactin and reported that it was effective against Gram-positive bacteria including *S. aureus*, as well as *Mycobacterium tuberculosis*.[8] It appeared to belong to a new class of antibiotics, which they say suggests that this approach could also yield more antibiotics that are different enough from what we already have to be truly useful.

Teixobactin is currently still in preclinical development. It will have to go through further testing before it can start to be considered as an antibiotic drug in humans, but for Lewis and Epstein it was a proof of concept for how we may be able to use new methods to delve deeper into the microbial world around us.

Designer antimicrobials

Another reason it's so hard to discover new kinds of antimicrobials is that it's difficult to search for something that's entirely unknown. How can you find something when you don't know what you're looking for?

One suggestion is to use artificial intelligence (AI). Jim Collins, Termeer professor of medical engineering and science at MIT, runs a lab that is using AI to try to discover new antibiotics. He and his team have used a deep neural network – an AI model inspired by the human brain – to try to spot molecules that may have antibiotic properties.

To do this, they put together a training set of around 2,500 compounds and tested these against *E. coli* bacteria to see which ones had an antibacterial effect. They then trained the neural network on this data; it was given information about the structure of each compound, and whether that compound had successfully inhibited bacterial growth.

They then set the neural network on a fresh dataset comprising more than 6,000 different compounds from the Broad Institute's Drug Repurposing Hub, a library of compounds studied in relation to all kinds of diseases.

The idea was that the neural network could identify promising antibiotics from this library, based on what it had learned from the training data. The key distinction here is that Collins and his team didn't 'tell' the neural network to look for anything particular in the structure of the compounds it examined. They let the neural network figure out for itself which features might be associated with antibacterial activity. This means it could potentially find patterns that we humans miss.

Using this approach, Collins and his team identified an antibiotic compound they called halicin (after HAL 9000, the AI in the film *2001: A Space Odyssey*). Halicin, they reported in a 2020 paper in the journal *Cell*, shows activity against a broad range of bacteria.[9] In tests with mice, it has been shown to be effective against *Clostridioides difficile* and the Gram-negative bacterium *A. baumannii*, which is one of the WHO's top-priority pathogens for finding new antibiotics.[10]

Halicin, which was originally being pursued as a diabetes drug, is now being further investigated to see if it could become a useful antibiotic for humans, but Collins says the real promise is in the platform. This kind of 'in silico' approach – experimenting using a computer rather than test tubes and Petri dishes – could enable the analysis of huge numbers of molecules. Collins hopes it could even move beyond drug discovery and into drug design. 'Because the model is able to identify features of molecules that make for good antibiotics, that enables us now to design from the bottom up molecules with desired properties, including significant antibacterial activity,' he says. 'And thus we can both explore and even create new chemical space that didn't exist before.'

Collins sees AI as a complementary approach to traditional drug discovery methods. And for now at least, he doesn't see AI usurping human researchers' roles. Once the computer model has made its predictions about auspicious-looking molecules, it's still down to researchers to identify the most promising ones and put them through their paces. 'I think we're still at a stage where the most promising efforts in this space come from where machine intelligence is integrated with human intelligence,' he says.

The real work begins

Discovering a potential new antibiotic substance is just the start. Next comes development: turning it into an actual drug. 'That's when the process gets expensive and takes time,' says the University of Plymouth's Mathew Upton.

First, you need to purify the compound and analyse its chemistry. You also need to check that it's not toxic. This is done by screening the compound against human or animal cells. 'It might be [that] you've got a compound which is really potent and kills all the sorts of bacteria that you want to kill, but it's also quite toxic to human cells,' Upton says. In which case, you either have to give up, or see if there's a way to tweak the chemistry to make it non-toxic to humans, without also reducing the antimicrobial activity.

The compound then needs to be subjected to a strict series of preclinical trials before it can advance to clinical trials (the first time it's tested in humans) – first to check it's safe, and then to check it's effective. It's a process that takes years, and the majority of promising compounds won't make it. 'From 10,000 things that look interesting on your first plate screen, you may get one thing that makes it to the clinic,' Upton estimates.

It's not just a science problem. One of the major hurdles to discovering and developing new antimicrobials is money. Often, despite the desperate need to find new antimicrobials, it just doesn't make financial sense.

This is something that Kevin Outterson, a professor of law at Boston University and executive director of the non-profit CARB-X, is trying to address. Outterson wrote his first major academic paper on balancing innovation and access in the prescription drug markets.[11] It was, as he describes, a '90-page, dense, law professor sort of article' considering the impacts of drug prices. But as he wrote it, he realised there was a big asterisk to his overall findings: some of the core assumptions about how the market works just don't hold true for antimicrobials.

If you make a drug to tackle cancer, or heart disease, or Alzheimer's, it will likely be instantly popular and will continue to be in demand through generations. But that's not necessarily the case for antimicrobials. Firstly, while we know that we will need new antimicrobials, it's hard to predict when exactly a specific existing antimicrobial will lose efficacy owing to emerging resistance – so it's hard to know when we will need a replacement. But by the time those existing drugs do become ineffective, it's too late to start developing a new one from scratch, and so we need to have a backup already in the arsenal. This means, however, that we need pharmaceutical companies to develop drugs that may not immediately be in high demand. 'This timing issue means that, when a novel new antibiotic reaches the market, we may not need it on a mass basis yet,' Outterson says.

This is compounded by the issue of resistance. The more a drug is used, the more likely resistance is to emerge. So as soon as a new antimicrobial drug becomes available, we will want to use it as little as possible in order to prevent resistance from emerging against it. We want to save new antimicrobial drugs for use only when existing ones fail, holding them in reserve as a safety net. This is good for public health, but bad for drug makers. We're effectively asking people to develop drugs so that we can *not* use them wherever possible. As a result, many of the largest pharmaceutical companies and investors have moved away from developing antimicrobials.

Outterson couldn't get this problem out of his mind, so in 2016 he co-founded CARB-X (which stands for Combating Antibiotic-Resistant Bacteria Biopharmaceutical Accelerator). CARB-X is funded by the UK, US and German governments, as well as the Wellcome Trust and the Bill & Melinda Gates Foundation. Its mission is to identify and fund the small companies and research groups working on the most promising, innovative antimicrobials, and other products that may help address antimicrobial resistance. It's stepping into the shoes previously filled by private investors, to try to keep antimicrobial innovation flowing. 'Our goal is to get them to the point where they've completed their first human trials and are ready for a couple of other programmes to pick them up and bring them across the finish line,' Outterson says. 'But we're here mainly because the market for innovation is broken.'

CARB-X has funded 92 projects, with a focus on the WHO's priority pathogens and the most innovative techniques; the idea is to find whole new antibiotic classes, not drugs similar to those we already have. Outterson predicts that CARB-X's efforts will result in two new antibiotics reaching the market in the next ten years. But, he says, it's impossible to predict how many, or which, products we may need, and by when. 'We don't know for sure whether our efforts are big enough, or should be five times bigger,' he says.

Ultimately, it would be better if new business models could incentivise pharmaceutical companies to push research in the antimicrobial space, so that projects like

CARB-X aren't as necessary. Here, the UK is taking a lead. The NHS is piloting a world-first subscription scheme for antimicrobials, where companies are paid upfront for access to their product, rather than when it is used in a patient.[12] It's a way of delinking the price paid for a new antimicrobial from the volumes used – like a subscription. Some refer to it as a 'Netflix model' for antibiotics. The idea is to recognise that the number of people using an antimicrobial does not necessarily reflect its value to the healthcare system; the most important antimicrobials could be those that are only used in a few extreme cases where nothing else works.

In 2020, the NHS, alongside the National Institute for Health and Care Excellence (NICE) and the Department of Health and Social Care (DHSC), selected the first two drugs to trial this payment model with: Zavicefta, a combination antimicrobial made by Pfizer that is licensed to treat infections including UTIs and hospital-acquired pneumonia, and Fetcroja, made by Japanese pharmaceutical company Shionogi and used to treat some Gram-negative infections.[13] NICE will evaluate the products and decide how much to pay to 'subscribe' for access to them. In the US, the proposed PASTEUR Act (the Pioneering Antimicrobial Subscriptions to End Upsurging Resistance Act) suggests a similar model, with drug developers paid on a subscription basis.[14]

Outterson hopes that one day he'll be out of a job because CARB-X won't be needed. Funding innovations such as subscription models would incentivise private investors once again to put money into antimicrobial discovery and development. Really, he says, it makes sense to pay upfront. He compares investment in antimicrobials to fire safety: imagine if we waited for a fire to break out before installing sprinklers, training firefighters or designing fire engines? It is far better to pay for protective measures so they're there when we need them.

***

Technological and conceptual advances in how to discover and develop new antimicrobials mean that there's lots to be hopeful about. But when we find new antimicrobials, we need to be careful how we use them. Continued overuse and misuse may lead to resistance emerging to those new drugs too, and it's likely that for as long as we keep finding new antimicrobials, we'll also keep finding new examples of antimicrobial resistance.

This makes it all the more important to use new antimicrobials wisely, so we can hold off resistance for as long as possible. And we can't stop once we've developed the next generation; the search for new antimicrobials must continue. 'Unless we find something that is completely game-changing, we are going to be continually needing to carry on looking,' Upton says.

4

Diagnostics and surveillance

More than three centuries ago, in 1714, the British government announced a series of prizes for anyone who could work out how to solve a problem that had long imperilled those voyaging at sea: calculating longitude. Working out latitude was easy enough, but an inability to accurately measure a ship's position from east to west made sailing a dangerous activity.[1] To incentivise innovation, the government passed the Longitude Act, which offered rewards of up to £20,000 (equivalent to several million pounds today) to any person who could develop a method of measuring longitude while at sea within a certain accuracy. Several inventors were awarded prizes, with clockmaker John Harrison ultimately taking the largest sum for his invention of a marine chronometer.

But what does this have to do with antimicrobial resistance? In 2014, inspired by this 300-year-old prize, UK innovation charity Nesta came up with a new one. It wanted to use the same idea of a financial incentive to solve one of the day's biggest scientific challenges. A public vote decided that antibiotics should be the focus. So it was that the twenty-first-century Longitude Prize – nothing to do with seafaring – put out a call for innovators to develop a test for bacterial infections. The test had to be fast, accurate, affordable and easy to use, with the overall winner in line for an £8 million reward.

Diagnostic tools are a critical part of the antimicrobial resistance puzzle. While we desperately need new antimicrobials, there's an obvious problem: as soon as we start to use these drugs, we risk resistance emerging to them, too. To prevent this as much as possible, we need to be better about only deploying antimicrobials when they are really necessary. New testing and diagnostics technology could help us turn a corner. Faster and more accurate diagnoses would allow clinicians to be more targeted in which drugs they prescribe and under which circumstances. This could help rein in some of the over-use and misuse that fuels resistance, while also making sure that patients receive the best treatment.

Competitors in the Longitude Prize come from all over the world and are targeting an array of different pathogens and infections, using different technologies. One team is Mologic, a UK-based social enterprise that makes diagnostic tech, including lateral flow tests for Covid-19. Its Longitude entry focuses on detecting sepsis. Sepsis isn't actually an infection *per se*; it's caused by the body's own immune system launching a severe reaction to an infection, especially in the bloodstream. It's a serious condition: sepsis kills 11 million people worldwide each year, many of whom are children. That's about one in five annual deaths globally that are caused by sepsis.[2]

Mologic's test is a lateral flow test, similar to a pregnancy test or the home tests you may be familiar with for Covid-19. A clinician takes a finger-prick of a patient's blood and puts it on the test. The test is then inserted into a reader, which analyses the results and tells the clinician whether the sample tests positive for so-called 'biomarkers' of sepsis or not, all within 20 minutes.

Emily Adams, Mologic's director of epidemics and neglected tropical diseases, says that it's hard to develop a lateral flow test for sepsis as bacteria are only present at very low levels in the blood. For this reason, Mologic's test is not actually looking to detect bacteria; it is instead measuring the body's own response by looking for a group of features – biomarkers – in the blood sample that may be associated with sepsis.

To develop the test, Adams explains that the company used machine-learning algorithms to identify the relative levels of different biomarkers associated with sepsis. It then ran a clinical trial on patients to check if the resulting model accurately caught those who went on to have confirmed sepsis, based on these relative biomarker levels.

The lateral flow test is looking for these biomarkers. The idea is to make sure that antibiotics are prescribed judiciously, 'so only people that absolutely require antibiotics will be given them, and those that don't will not have wastage or overusage of antibiotics, which allows resistance to proliferate,' Adams says.

It will be at least a couple of years before Mologic's test is ready for use in hospitals and clinics, after which point it will be important to observe how it works in practice – for example, how it actually influences clinicians' decisions about patient care. The thing is that tests can't always give a yes-or-no answer. It's not possible for a test to say with certainty whether a given person really needs antibiotics or not; a clinician needs to make that call. 'There's a real sort of grey area in between, where people may require them; they *might* be beneficial,' Adams says. Doctors may be risk-averse, and choosing *not* to prescribe antibiotics, even as a just-in-case, could be a tough decision – in which case they could continue to prescribe the drugs anyway. 'We're [ideally] going to need randomised controlled trials to really prove that the technology hasan impact on patient outcome,' Adams says.

Testing for resistance

In the case of sepsis, which can quickly become deadly, detecting an infection quickly is paramount. But in some situations, just knowing whether someone has a bacterial infection or not may not be so helpful when it comes to deciding how to treat them. In fact, it could inadvertently lead to more antibiotic prescribing. This is because not everyone who has a bacterial infection actually needs antibiotics to get rid of it; they might be able to fight it off on their own. Someone with mild symptoms, even if they are caused by an infection, may be better advised to rest up and take some paracetamol, and let their immune system take care of it. But if clinicians are faced with a test result that confirms the presence of a pathogen, they may be swayed to prescribe antibiotics where previously they might have waited.

Because of this, approaches to the Longitude Prize have evolved since its inception. The key question now, says Daniel Berman, director of global health and disability at Nesta Challenges, is not just whether a bacterial infection is present. 'Now, the question is, what is the bug? Or what class of bug? And then which antibiotic will work?' he says.

Currently, it can take days for clinicians to find out which microbe is causing an infection, and whether it has resistance to any particular antimicrobial. The standard testing method is pretty old-school: a sample, such as blood or urine, is taken from the patient and sent to the lab. Here, it's placed on a plate of agar and any microbes present are left to grow. The microbiologist can then examine the microbial colonies to identify the troublesome bug, or bugs. They can test for antibiotic resistance by putting a small amount of antibiotics on the plate with the microbe. If the microbe doesn't grow around an antibiotic, it's susceptible – the antimicrobial works. But if the microbe happily grows, unbothered by the presence of the antibiotic, it's resistant.

Often, doctors will prescribe a broad-spectrum antibiotic, or a best guess, while they wait for results – if they do a test at all. It can be quicker and cheaper just to prescribe whichever antimicrobial usually works, and only investigate further if symptoms don't resolve. Patients, too, may be reluctant to wait days for treatment when they could be cured by the time results come in if a doctor would just give them a prescription on their first visit. And in some cases, it's too dangerous to wait; clinicians don't have a choice but to administer their best-bet antimicrobials and hope that they work.

Some Longitude Prize teams are attempting to develop diagnostic tools that can identify microbes more quickly. Module Innovations, based in Pune, India, is working on diagnostic tools for urinary tract infections (UTIs). UTIs are one of the most common infections, especially in women, with an estimated 150 million occurring every year.[3] While they are often easily treated, if not diagnosed or managed properly they can develop into kidney or even bloodstream infections – not to mention they can be painful and debilitating.

Sometimes, a clinician may collect a sample of urine to test for a UTI. But because they will often also prescribe a broad-spectrum antibiotic to treat the symptoms straight away, the patient may have already finished their prescription by the time the results come back. Hopefully, the test confirms that they took a suitable drug; if not, they may need to take another – and their infection may have got worse in the meantime. Other patients may present with UTI-like symptoms that are actually not caused by an infection, meaning antibiotics aren't an appropriate treatment.

Module Innovations co-founder and CEO Sachin Dubey says he recognised the need for a better UTI test after a family member got a UTI while she was pregnant. She was given a broad-spectrum antibiotic that didn't work well for her and had to wait days for the pathogen to be identified and the correct antibiotic to be prescribed. 'So during her pregnancy, she had to suffer a lot,' he says.

Module Innovations is working on two products that target different parts of the healthcare system. One, designed to enable doctors to prescribe antibiotics more accurately, is a credit-card-sized lateral flow test called USense. It can tell within around 15 minutes whether a urine sample contains an infection-causing bacteria, and also whether the bacteria is Gram-negative or Gram-positive. A second diagnostic device, called ASTSense, goes a step further. The size of a small printer, it aims to identify antibiotic resistance in the bacteria (AST stands for antibiotic susceptibility testing). The principle behind ASTSense is similar to that of a standard bacterial culture: the urine sample is tested against a panel of different antibiotics, and whether the bacteria grows or not reveals which antibiotics it has resistance to. But where Module Innovations claims to offer an advantage over traditional tests is that it can deliver results in two hours rather than two days, owing to nanoprobes it has developed that the company says allow the growth of the bacteria to be detected more quickly.

The diagnostics are still being validated, but Dubey envisions a world where a patient could present to a doctor with a suspected UTI, find out in 15 minutes whether an infection is actually present, and then get a message a couple of hours later telling them which antibiotic to take. This way, patients could receive the most appropriate treatment right away, and doctors could prescribe antimicrobials in a more targeted manner.

There are many other competitors in the Longitude Prize, which will soon be drawing to a close. The winning diagnostic will be decided according to seven criteria: it must be needed, accurate, affordable, rapid, easy-to-use, safe and scalable. A panel of expert judges will help to interpret these measures as they apply to each test. But while there will be one main winner, the real objective of the Longitude Prize is to foster an ecosystem of people who are all working on the issue. 'We feel like it's been a success in the sense of mobilising new technologies towards a certain problem,' Berman says. The Prize has attracted more than 250 competitors in total, with around 50 making it through to the last stages. The final deadline for entries will be in September 2022.

Other groups around the world are also turning their attention to the same cause. In 2019, a company called Visby Medical won the US-based Antimicrobial Resistance Diagnostic Challenge, taking a prize of $19 million for its rapid test for gonorrhoea.[4] WHO data shows that drug-resistant gonorrhoea is on the rise, with many countries reporting strains resistant to common antibiotics such as ciprofloxacin. In 2018, Public Health England (PHE) reported on the first global case of gonorrhoea resistant to the usual first-line drugs plus many other antibiotics. The patient was ultimately able to be treated, but PHE warned that 'identifying treatment options for the case was challenging as few remained'.[5]

Visby Medical's device aims to identify whether the *Neisseria gonorrhoeae* bacteria causing an infection are resistant to ciprofloxacin within 30 minutes. To do this, it detects a change in a gene, known as a single nucleotide polymorphism (SNP), that confers resistance to ciprofloxacin, using PCR testing (you may have come across PCR testing if you ever had to go for a Covid-19 test, except in this case the samples come from genital rather than nasal swabs). It's an example of 'genotype' testing – looking at the genetic properties of the pathogen – as opposed to 'phenotype' testing, which looks at its observable characteristics. Sequencing the full DNA of a microbe is time-consuming and expensive, but methods like this can offer an insight into relevant bits of the genome without the need to sequence it all. Visby hopes to add its test for ciprofloxacin resistance into a diagnostic device aimed at women's sexual health, which will test for gonorrhoea as well as chlamydia and trichomoniasis, two other sexually transmitted infections.[6]

Gary Schoolnik, a professor of medicine at Stanford University and chief medical officer at Visby Medical, believes that using genotypic data will be crucial in our ongoing battle against antimicrobial resistance. The key is being able to get that information fast and make it affordable to deploy. Testing for resistance in this way, he says, could 'have a huge effect on limiting antimicrobial resistance, because we won't be using antibiotics where they don't have to be used, and we won't be using huge broad-spectrum antimicrobial regimens because we don't know what to treat a patient with'.

As with discovering new antimicrobial drugs, of course, the 'science part' is just the start when it comes to developing new tests. Making a diagnostic tool that is accurate and effective is one thing; getting it into widespread manufacturing and usage, where it can help steer antimicrobial use in the real world, is another. Here, financing can again be a barrier. Many first-line antibiotic drugs are very cheap – cheaper than conducting a test. Encouraging health services to invest in testing will require convincing them of its value and allocating sufficient resources.

Surveillance

Information gathered from diagnostic tests can help get the right treatment to an individual patient, but it can also feed into a broader picture of infectious disease and resistance. When you start pooling data, you can glean useful insights into how pathogens are spreading and how resistance is evolving on a larger scale. This kind of surveillance is important; after all, you can't hope to find solutions without knowing the shape and extent of the problem.

In 2015, the WHO launched the Global Antimicrobial Resistance and Use Surveillance System (GLASS) with the aim of standardising the collection, analysis and sharing of data related to antimicrobial resistance around the world. Its routine data surveillance programme, GLASS-AMR, focuses on eight priority pathogens: *Acinetobacter, E. coli, Klebsiella pneumoniae, Neisseria gonorrhoeae, Salmonella, Shigella, Staphylococcus aureus* and *Streptococcus pneumoniae*.[7] When samples are taken from patients and tested for clinical purposes, the results – which may show which pathogens are present and which drugs they are resistant to – can also be added into the datasets of surveillance programmes like GLASS to build up a picture of resistance in that location and beyond. The most recent GLASS-AMR report, published in 2021, is informed by data collected across 70 countries, concerning a total of more than 3 million laboratory-confirmed infections.[8]

This kind of data surveillance can help to answer some basic questions, such as how extensive the burden of antimicrobial resistance is. It can also flag patterns of resistance in a particular geography or among a particular demographic, and spot emerging resistance before it becomes widespread. Insights from the data can be used to help influence policy, direct research activities and inform prevention and control efforts.

'Surveillance is one of the key pillars of understanding and combating antimicrobial resistance,' says Nicholas Feasey, a professor at Liverpool School of Tropical Medicine who is currently based at the Malawi Liverpool Wellcome Trust Clinical Research Programme in Blantyre, Malawi. To take an example from his own work, Feasey says that routine bacteriological surveillance at Queen

Elizabeth Central Hospital in Blantyre alerted him and his colleagues to a rapid increase in a multidrug-resistant strain of *Salmonella typhi*, the bacteria that causes typhoid fever.[9] This observation was key in flagging the re-emergence of typhoid fever as a major problem in the area, and the city was subsequently selected to be part of a trial of a new typhoid vaccine funded by the Bill & Melinda Gates Foundation, with promising results.[10]

'It is so impactful to be able to show people data from their setting,' Feasey says. He is also principal investigator of the Drivers of Resistance in Uganda and Malawi (DRUM) consortium, which found that 70 per cent of river water samples in Blantyre contained a type of *E. coli* known as extended-spectrum beta-lactamase (ESBL) *E. coli*. ESBLs are a type of enzyme produced by bacteria that make some antibiotics (the beta-lactam antibiotics, which include penicillins) ineffective. The implication: the river water was full of drug-resistant *E. coli*. When Feasey presented the data to people working on antimicrobial resistance at the Malawi Ministry of Health, he says there were audible gasps; they were horrified. 'So surveillance data have the ability to be incredibly impactful when communicating with policymakers,' he says.

Surveillance can be challenging, however, particularly at an international scale. First, you need to be able to collect trustworthy data, which may be harder in lower-resource settings. Analysing samples requires trained staff, a consistent supply of materials and sufficient facilities, including electricity and a reliable cold chain (i.e. the ability to keep necessary items refrigerated during transportation and storage). In order to make sense of differences across countries, there also has to be standardisation as to how data is collected, so that meaningful comparisons can be drawn. The recent WHO GLASS-AMR report, for instance, raised concerns that there were much higher reported rates in bloodstream infections caused by resistant *E. coli* and MRSA in low- and middle-income countries than in high-income countries.[11] This could suggest that lower-income countries are more affected by resistance, but it could also mean that the data has been subject to selection bias (or both things may be true). If fewer people are tested in lower-income countries – perhaps because of greater pressure on resources – then a higher proportion of samples may show resistance, because testing is reserved for the most problematic cases. If you're only sampling people after they've already tried several different antibiotics, for instance, then you're likely to find a higher proportion of resistant infections.

There's also the technical problem of how to handle such vast quantities of data in a way that is most useful. Ideally, you want a data management system that can get test results to a patient in good time, while also feeding into national surveillance systems and global repositories such as GLASS. And this all needs to happen without putting too much burden on clinicians as they go about their work helping patients. 'Really, to make sense of the burden of drug-resistant infection, we need to think more deeply about what is the minimum amount of data we need to inform global surveillance parameters, and what is the maximum amount of data that is acceptable to a junior doctor at four o'clock in the morning to put on a specimen form,' Feasey says.

The secrets of the genome

If you want to really know what's going on inside bacteria, you need to look closer than through a microscope at an agar plate. Genome sequencing can unravel the secrets written in bacterial DNA.

A quick refresher: DNA is made up of two strands in the form of a double helix. These strands are made up of four bases, represented by the letters A, C, G and T, which pair up to connect the two strands. The sequence of these bases within a portion of DNA – a gene – makes up the genetic code that instructs a cell in which proteins to make.

If you sequence the genome of bacteria, you can look for genes or mutations known to be associated with antimicrobial resistance. This can help to determine which antimicrobial to prescribe to someone who has a resistant infection, as in Visby Medical's gonorrhoea test. But further magic happens when you look at the bigger picture and apply genome sequencing to surveillance.

'Genomics has quite a unique role to play in understanding and tracking antimicrobial resistance, because it tells us what is actually spreading in a way that no other technology can do,' says Kathryn Holt, professor of microbial systems genomics at the London School of Hygiene and Tropical Medicine and co-director of its Antimicrobial Resistance Centre. Sequence a microbe's genome and you won't just find out which pathogen it is or whether it is resistant to a particular drug; you can also identify which mechanisms of resistance it has (i.e. how it escapes the drug's effects) and get insight into how it is spreading.

Say you have two patients presenting with an infection. If a bacterium sampled from person A is genetically very similar to one sampled from person B, you may be able to determine that A has picked it up from B, or vice versa. On a larger scale, you might find a cluster of patients with the same strain of bacteria and be able to track the spread within a hospital ward, healthcare facility or community, or even between countries. We saw genomic data used this way during the Covid-19 pandemic in detecting different variants of the virus: alpha, beta, gamma, delta and so on. It's the same virus, SARS-CoV-2, but with different variants, distinguishable by genome sequencing, which can be associated with different features such as greater transmissibility or lower severity of illness.

Labs that conduct genome sequencing in the context of antimicrobial resistance can use the data to try to spot trends, so that clinicians and policymakers can take steps to prevent outbreaks of particularly troublesome resistant pathogens. Holt gives the example of a cluster of infections caused by resistant bacteria on a hospital ward: other people on the ward could be screened to see if they are colonised by the same resistant bug and given treatment before they get sick. 'The earlier you can detect that chain of transmission and break it, the more infections you save,' she says. Other actions could include changing the antimicrobial used to treat a particular type of infection if resistance levels to the current first-line treatment are increasing, and stepping up infection control methods.

Genomics could also help researchers to spot new forms of drug-resistant outbreaks. Take shigellosis. Caused by the *Shigella* genus of bacteria, shigellosis is an infection that results in diarrhoea, fever and pain, and is best known for causing dysentery in lower-income countries. In England, infections in adults have historically tended to be linked to overseas travel, but in recent years public health officials have noticed an increase in cases specifically among gay and bisexual men. Among these cases, antibiotic resistance is very common.[12] Genome sequencing was able to show links between cases of shigellosis, helping to spot 'clusters' of infection among men who have sex with men – and likely representing sexual transmission.[13] 'That changed the general understanding of the epidemiology

SUPERBUGS

of shigellosis in England,' Holt explains. 'It led to the recognition of that particular kind of infection as a sexually transmitted infection.'

This kind of insight can inform public health activities, helping clinicians and officials to target services where they are most needed. In this case, it meant increasing awareness about shigellosis among gay and bisexual men, directing resources to sexual health clinics, and advising clinicians on prescribing practices considering the high prevalence of resistance to certain antimicrobials. It's urgent work: at the beginning of 2022, the UK Health Security Agency reported a rise in cases of 'extremely antibiotic-resistant' sexually transmitted *Shigella* infections.[14]

There are many other things that genomic data might also shed light on. It could, for instance, help to flag where resistant bacteria are transferring to humans from animals, or help to detect resistant bacteria in the environment. Sequencing samples of wastewater, for example, could give an insight into concerning bugs circulating in the community before they start hitting hospitals.

David Aanensen, director of the Centre for Genomic Pathogen Surveillance at the University of Oxford's Big Data Institute, foresees a time when anyone who presents to a hospital with an infection will have a sample sent off for sequencing, which could then be used both as a diagnostic tool and as information that feeds back into broader surveillance systems. 'Genomics is a leap forward, because you can replace a lot of laboratory techniques by looking at the genome,' he says.

At the moment, there are a few different sequencing platforms out there. Most public health labs use Illumina sequencers, which sequence fragments of DNA. Another technology, known as nanopore sequencing, is also generating interest, as it is able to more rapidly sequence DNA at low cost. One exciting advance, says Holt, involves sequencing DNA directly from a specimen – a sputum, urine or blood sample – rather than having to culture the microbe in a Petri dish first. 'Skipping the culture step could potentially take us from getting answers in two days to getting answers in about two hours,' she says.

That's not to say that there aren't challenges. Genome sequencing is still relatively expensive, so even when the technology has been perfected, there will be a challenge to get it integrated into healthcare settings, particularly in low- and middle-income countries. And much also depends on creating a data infrastructure that can make the most of any data collected, both locally and globally. Aanensen points out that, even in high-income countries, GPs still sometimes use paper health records – not exactly conducive to large-scale data sharing. Part of his work is focused on democratising access to genome data by creating visualisations that make it easy for people to compare and interpret their findings. 'The future is being able to see the reporting from these strings of ACTGs come alive, and contextualising the data you put in with everything else in the world right there and then,' he says.

***

The more knowledge we have about antimicrobial resistance, the better prepared we will be to defend against it. Diagnostic tools that can identify pathogens will help us to better manage our use of antimicrobials, resulting in more targeted treatments for patients while reducing unnecessary antimicrobial consumption. Meanwhile, large-scale surveillance will allow us to keep tabs on emerging resistance so that we can adapt our response as needed. It will help us to track even basic facts, such as how many people are affected by antimicrobial resistance, and which microbes and resistance mechanisms pose the largest threat. Only by understanding what we're up against can we truly work to tackle it.

5

Antibiotic alternatives

As resistance to antimicrobials (and particularly antibiotics) grows, might it not be better to try something different? While we're unlikely ever to find a silver bullet for infectious disease, there are other approaches that could have a role in tackling antimicrobial resistance, most likely as a complement to antibiotics rather than a replacement.

Bacterial vaccines

As Covid-19 became officially recognised as a pandemic towards the start of 2020, hopes were pinned on one particular solution: a vaccine. A preventative tool rather than a treatment, vaccines work by priming the body's immune system to fight off an infectious disease by itself.

Here's a reminder of the basics: a pathogen, such as a disease-causing bacterium or virus, has specific proteins on its surface known as antigens. When the pathogen infects the body, the immune system makes antibodies that fight against specific antigens, but it can take a while to produce these. A vaccine effectively exposes the immune system to parts of the antigen in a safe way, so that it starts producing the relevant antibodies without the person becoming infected. If that person is later exposed to the real antigen, the immune system can more rapidly produce the antibodies needed to fight it, thanks to 'memory cells' that draw on their previous experience with the antigen in question.[1] As a result, vaccines can prevent an infection from taking hold in the first place, or can save a person from experiencing the most severe symptoms.

Vaccines are a crucial tool in tackling antimicrobial resistance. By reducing the transmission of an infectious disease overall, you naturally also reduce the transmission of resistant infections; fewer people get sick, and fewer people spread resistant bugs. Vaccination also reduces the need to use antimicrobial drugs, as if people's immune systems are able to fight off a pathogen themselves then they don't need to take antimicrobials – which means the microbes aren't exposed to the selective pressure applied by antimicrobials, which is a driver of resistance. 'As the level of those pathogens decreases, obviously the number of bacteria with antimicrobial resistance decreases, but also the amount of disease that's being caused by those bacterial pathogens reduces, and the use of antibiotics reduces, so you then get into a positive cycle that can reduce antimicrobial resistance,' explains Cal MacLennan, a clinician and immunologist whose titles include senior programme officer for bacterial vaccines at the Gates Foundation, senior clinical fellow at the Jenner Institute in Oxford, and director of the BactiVac network at the University of Birmingham.

But while multiple vaccines were developed for Covid-19 in a matter of months, vaccines that work against bacterial infections can be tricky. One reason for this is that bacteria are just more complex than viruses. Most Covid-19 vaccines, for instance, aim for the 'spike protein' found on the surface of the SARS-CoV-2 virus, but bacteria generally don't have such a juicy target. And while we've seen great innovation in the development of Covid-19 vaccines, such as mRNA vaccines and viral vector vaccines, 'those aren't so easily applicable to bacteria, where you're dealing with a much more complex pathogen,' MacLennan says. (Of course, some viruses are also difficult to make a vaccine for; HIV poses a particular challenge, partly because it mutates so rapidly.)

We do routinely vaccinate against certain bacterial diseases, especially in children. Some bacterial vaccines work by using a killed or weakened form of the relevant bacteria. Vaccines for tetanus and diphtheria work by targeting the toxins produced by the bacteria, rather than the bacteria themselves. The Hib (*Haemophilus influenzae*

B) vaccine, pneumococcal conjugate vaccine and several meningococcal vaccines are examples of 'conjugate' vaccines,[2] which usually work by invoking an immune response to the capsule that surrounds the bacterial cell. (This approach doesn't work for all bacteria, however, because they don't all have capsules.)

In his role at the Gates Foundation, MacLennan is working on vaccines for *Salmonella* and *Shigella*, two types of bacteria that cause gastrointestinal infections and lead to the deaths of hundreds of thousands of young children every year.[3] Various approaches are being explored for vaccines that might defend against these bacteria. 'Covid has changed things hugely for viral vaccines going forward,' he says. 'We could really do with a similar breakthrough for bacterial vaccines.' Part of the problem, he adds, is that there has been little commercial incentive to develop vaccines for diseases that mainly affect low- and middle-income countries.

Meanwhile, at the Jenner Institute, MacLennan is leading a team developing a vaccine to prevent gonorrhoea. While gonorrhoea might not be that deadly, it is very prevalent; the WHO estimates that in 2016 there were 87 million new cases globally.[4] It's also a particular problem when it comes to antimicrobial resistance, to the point that the WHO warns we may start to see infections that are simply untreatable. Here, MacLennan and his team are trying to make a vaccine using 'outer membrane vesicles' – blobs on the outside of the *Neisseria gonorrhoeae* bacteria, which causes gonorrhoea – in order to provoke an immune response.[5] They hope that their vaccine will prevent people from getting the disease, and therefore prevent the spread of antimicrobial resistance, too.

Many other research groups and companies are also working on bacterial vaccines, focusing on different pathogens and using different approaches. Jan Poolman, vice-president and head of bacterial vaccine research and development at pharmaceutical company Janssen, previously worked on efforts to develop bacterial vaccines for babies and children at GSK. Now, he says, he's focused on 'the other spectrum of life where the immune system is suboptimal' – older people. His team is working on vaccines for *E. coli* and *Staphylococcus aureus*, which are the most common bacteria to cause sepsis. 'Those are the two lead bacteria that we are focusing on, because we want to prevent the most life-threatening forms of bacterial diseases in adults,' he says.

Poolman envisions that one day we could see universal vaccine programmes in adults for bacteria such as *E. coli* and *S. aureus*, just as there are for children to safeguard them from whooping cough or meningitis. An additional advantage of this approach could be the herd effect: if enough people are immunised, then even those who are not vaccinated may gain protection, as the bacteria has less opportunity to spread. For other vaccines, it may make more sense to target them to particular groups of people that are most vulnerable.

However, it may never be possible to create vaccines for all bacterial diseases. Poolman highlights mucosal infections, which can include UTIs, skin infections and respiratory infections, as a particular challenge. It could be hugely beneficial from an antimicrobial resistance perspective to vaccinate against these kinds of infections, as they drive a lot of antimicrobial consumption. Their nature, however, makes developing vaccines against them difficult, as the bacteria can hide in the body's tissues where they're harder to reach.

In addition, the business model for vaccines can pose a challenge. Firstly, developing a vaccine is very expensive. It's also time-consuming. The year that it took for the Covid-19 vaccines to be developed and rolled out is highly unusual; ten years is the more common timeframe. Testing vaccines is difficult, because their preventative nature means it is necessary to involve large numbers of healthy participants to see if any of them happen to get sick after being vaccinated. The upfront investment, says Poolman, means it's 'certainly not doable for smaller companies – essentially impossible'.

Nevertheless, vaccines are a crucial part of the antimicrobial resistance puzzle, and not just in humans, either. Vaccines for livestock can also mean a reduction in the use of antibiotics, relieving some of the selective pressure caused by widespread antibiotic use. There are even vaccines for fish: Norway has drastically reduced its use of antibiotics in salmon by using vaccines against bacterial diseases that affect fish, such as furunculosis.[6]

There's an increasing realisation, MacLennan says, that vaccines can have a major role in reducing antimicrobial resistance. Poolman quotes Benjamin Franklin: 'An ounce of prevention is worth a pound of cure.'

Monoclonal antibodies

Prevention may be preferable to cure, but sometimes we don't have a choice. Once you're already sick, treatment is the only option. Where vaccines prime our immune system as a preventative measure, monoclonal antibodies take our own natural immune response as the starting point for a potential treatment option, too.

To recap, antibodies are proteins that the body produces to identify and fight foreign bodies, such as infection-causing microbes. They do this by attaching themselves to the invader's antigens, thereby preventing it from doing damage.[7] Monoclonal antibodies are lab-produced biomolecules that take inspiration from this natural phenomenon. They can be injected into the skin or muscle, or be delivered intravenously into a patient's body, where they effectively take on the same role as a person's own antibodies, locating and binding to specific antigens.

'They mimic what the natural body would do when under attack, at a larger scale,' says Ayesha Sitlani, associate vice-president of antibody strategy at IAVI, the International AIDS Vaccine Initiative, which is calling for greater access to monoclonal antibodies for a broad range of diseases.[8] Monoclonal antibodies can help fight off pathogens before the immune system has had a chance to put up a strong defence, and could be particularly helpful for people who are immunocompromised and struggle to mount an immune response.

To date, monoclonal antibody-based treatments have largely been targeted at non-communicable diseases (i.e., ones that aren't transmitted from person to person), such as cancers and autoimmune diseases, but there is growing recognition that they could also play a role in treating infectious diseases, and especially those caused by drug-resistant microbes. The Covid-19 pandemic has also inspired a lot of interest in monoclonal antibodies, with many companies working on monoclonal antibody treatments against the virus.

Monoclonal antibodies could have several benefits over traditional antibiotics. They can target specific antigens, unlike broad-spectrum antimicrobials, and may have fewer side-effects. And because they can be designed to target specific types of protein – such as proteins that help the bacteria cause damage (known as virulence proteins) as opposed to proteins that the bacteria need for their own survival – they may lend themselves less to resistance, Sitlani says. This is because the proteins needed for survival tend to mutate most readily.

Sitlani foresees monoclonal antibodies being used to complement antibiotics, and in some cases perhaps replace them. A main hurdle at the moment is less on the research side and more on the business side. Cost is a real barrier, both to developing the treatments and then expanding access to them so that as many people as possible can benefit. A 2020 report by IAVI and Wellcome states that almost 80 per cent of sales of monoclonal antibodies are in the US, Canada and Europe, despite 85 per cent of the world's population living in low- and middle-income countries.[9] Innovations in producing and scaling up monoclonal antibodies will help to bring down the costs, but policy changes are also required. 'A lot of these monoclonal antibodies tend to be registered in high-income countries; their target product profiles [the frameworks used to design the products] are suited for high-income countries,' Sitlani says. 'But in order for these to reach all populations, and certainly populations that need them the most, the profiles need to be designed for delivery in those settings.'

Phage therapy

In 2015, Steffanie Strathdee, distinguished professor of medicine and associate dean of global health sciences at the University of California San Diego (UCSD), was confronted with an antimicrobial-resistant infection the likes of which she had never previously come across. The patient involved was a man who had developed pancreatitis, an inflammation of the pancreas, but further investigation revealed this was just the tip of the iceberg. A CT scan revealed a large pseudocyst – a sac inside the man's abdomen – that had likely been there for months. The pseudocyst had offered a perfect environment to harbour bacteria, and it had become home to a particularly nasty bug: a multidrug-resistant strain of *Acinetobacter baumannii*, a Gram-negative bacterium that tops the WHO's priority list of pathogens for which new antibiotics are critically needed.

In this case, the infection was resistant to almost all antibiotics, with just partial sensitivity to a few 'last-resort' drugs that are reserved for the most serious resistant infections and come with the risk of hefty side-effects. Faced with an infection that was rapidly getting worse, Strathdee was desperate to find a solution that might save the man's life. It was particularly crucial to her, because this wasn't just any patient. It was her husband.

Strathdee and her husband, Thomas Patterson, had been on holiday in Egypt when things had started to go wrong. They'd just enjoyed a final dinner on their trip, a romantic meal under the stars aboard a cruise ship on its way to Luxor, when Patterson had begun to feel unwell. He then vomited through the night. 'I just thought he had food poisoning, and I was a bit annoyed because he was keeping me up,' Strathdee says. But as the night turned to morning and Patterson's condition worsened, a trip to the local clinic resulted in the diagnosis of acute pancreatitis. Patterson was medevacked to Germany, where the pseudocyst was discovered – about the size of a football and full of murky brown liquid, indicative of a microbial infection. A sample was cultured, and the results were even more worrying: *A. baumannii*.

For Strathdee, the implications of the test results were not immediately apparent. An epidemiologist rather than a medical doctor, she recalled studying *A. baumannii* during her undergraduate microbiology training decades previously. Back then, she says, it was seen as a 'really wimpy organism'. But with antimicrobial resistance on the rise, *A. baumannii* has evolved into a much more dangerous threat. In the US, it has gained the nickname 'Iraqibacter' because of its prevalence among wounded soldiers who have picked up infections while serving in Iraq and other Middle Eastern countries.[10] The reason it is such an urgent threat is because it is particularly adept at gaining resistance via multiple mechanisms, including through plasmids, meaning many infections are multidrug resistant or even pandrug resistant.[11] 'I consider it something of a bacterial kleptomaniac,' Strathdee says. 'It's really great at stealing antimicrobial resistance genes from other bacteria and the environment.'

An antibiotic sensitivity test revealed that Patterson's infection was indeed highly drug-resistant. Patterson was ultimately medevacked back to San Diego, where he took up residence in the intensive care unit. In one sense, Strathdee and Patterson had everything on their side: they were back on home turf, and the leading experts treating Patterson's infection were not just colleagues but friends. Robert 'Chip' Schooley, head of infectious diseases at UCSD, had been offering advice from the onset of Patterson's illness, first over the phone and then in person on their return. Yet with the infection becoming resistant to all antibiotics, there was not much to be optimistic about. The pseudocyst was still there, and Patterson was now so frail that surgery was not an option; without any drugs in the arsenal, there was too great a risk that the infection could get into the bloodstream.

Over the course of several months, he kept getting sicker. One of the drains placed in his abdomen to remove infected fluid slipped, and the bacteria spread to his bloodstream, causing him to go into septic shock. After that, the bacteria were everywhere; he was fully colonised. His organs began to fail and he was in a coma. Strathdee could barely believe it: not so long ago he'd been climbing into pyramids and jumping onto boats, and now he was fighting for his life. 'I'm an infectious disease epidemiologist, so it was really like God's cruel joke,' she says.

With antibiotics offering no solution, Strathdee resolved to leave no stone unturned in trying to find a cure for her husband. 'I did what anybody would do,' she says. 'I hit the internet.'

It was while browsing results from the biomedical search engine PubMed that Strathdee came across an unconventional idea: bacteriophages. A bacteriophage (often just known as a phage) is a type of virus that infects bacteria but doesn't infect human cells. Once a phage has infected a bacterial cell, it effectively hijacks the cell's mechanisms to turn it into a phage-producing machine. The resulting phages eventually burst out of the cell, destroying it, in an action called lysis.[12]

It's an attractively simple idea: use a virus to infect the bacteria that are infecting a person. And it's by no means new. Bacteriophages were discovered in the early twentieth century and were even used to treat bacterial infections in the 1920s and 1930s, especially in the former USSR.[13] But with the discovery of antibiotics, bacteriophage research became largely forgotten, at least in the West. Antibiotics were so good at treating bacterial infections, and the early research around phages was not enough to convince many researchers to pursue them as a potential therapy. There was perhaps an element of geopolitical stigma that put off Western researchers, too: phages were still being used in the USSR, particularly in Georgia, where the Eliava Institute, an influential centre for bacteriophage therapy, was opened in 1923.

Strathdee found a paper referencing phage therapy in relation to *A. baumannii*,[14] but she couldn't find any record of it being used in humans. Nevertheless, she decided it had to be worth a shot.

One of the difficulties of phage therapy is that you need to match the right phage with the right microbe. Phages are found in the same places as the bacteria they feed on: in the environment and inside our own bodies. To find ones that might be effective against particularly nasty bugs, you need to look where you might also find those particularly nasty bugs – like in a festering swamp, or a sewage system. But phages can be picky: the team treating Patterson would not just need to find phages that worked against *A. baumannii* in general but ones that worked against the exact bacteria taken from his sample – his 'bacterial isolate'. And one phage wouldn't be enough; as with antibiotics, bacteria can evolve to defend themselves from phages, so it would be more effective to use a cocktail of different phages attacking from multiple angles. 'If you only have one phage, you're giving the bacteria a leg up to develop resistance to the phage,' Strathdee explains. Thus began a search for laboratories with phage libraries that might have one active against Patterson's infection.

Testing a phage is quite straightforward in principle. First, you take a sample of the bacteria from the infected person and grow it in the lab. Researchers then use something called a plaque assay: they take a Petri dish of agar and spread the bacteria over it, then add small drops of different phage solutions and let the whole thing incubate. The bacteria grow, forming an opaque layer. But in some places, it may appear to have small holes, like a slice of Emmental cheese. Here, the bacteria have been killed, leaving a small clearing or 'plaque' – and indicating that the phages placed on that spot have succeeded in infecting the bacteria. Researchers then test these promising phages further against the bacterial isolate.

With the assistance of many helpers, the UCSD team managed to identify several phages that showed promise. The full story, which involves several laboratories around the world, assistance from the US Navy, and a race to get permission to apply the phages under compassionate use, is detailed in Strathdee and Patterson's book, *The Perfect Predator: A Scientist's Race to Save Her Husband from a Deadly Superbug.*[15]

Just as difficult as finding the phages was then figuring out how to purify and administer them. Phages aren't a standard therapy by any means; there was no handy guide. They had little to go on in terms of dosage or how to apply them, but with Patterson by that point facing almost certain death without any intervention, they pushed ahead with the best regimen they could think of. 'We injected a billion phages per dose every two hours in his body, and it was the scariest day of my life when we did that, because it could have cured or killed him, nobody knew,' Strathdee says. (This dose was later reduced.)

A couple of days after treatment started, Patterson woke up from his coma. Against almost all expectations, the phage therapy had worked. 'One of the doctors described it as a Hail Mary pass in the last quarter of the football game, where the quarterback is blindfolded, throwing the ball over 100 yards down the field and hoping that somebody will catch it,' Strathdee recalls. 'And they did.'

Engineered phages

Patterson is a member of a very small club of people who have been treated with bacteriophages in this way. But since his recovery, there has been more interest in using phages when patients are out of other options.

Graham Hatfull, a professor of biological sciences at the University of Pittsburgh in Pennsylvania who studies phages, says he had never really been involved in therapeutic applications. He's not a physician or a clinician, but a 'nerdy basic biologist'. He is interested in characterising the genetic diversity of phages and works with thousands of students to isolate and catalogue them, with a focus on phages that infect a group of bacteria called mycobacteria. The *Mycobacterium* genus includes *Mycobacterium tuberculosis*, which causes TB, as well as many other species that are important to human health.

But, in 2017, Hatfull was contacted by James Soothill, a consultant microbiologist at Great Ormond Street Hospital in London, about a patient who was in a bad condition. The patient was a 15-year-old girl with cystic fibrosis who had been fighting an infection caused by drug-resistant *Mycobacterium abscessus*, which got worse after she had a double lung transplant (likely aided by the immunosuppressive medication needed to support the transplant). The wound from the transplant turned red and infected, and her body was covered in infected sores and nodules.[16] Standard treatments weren't working.

Prompted by the girl's mother, Soothill was considering the idea of phages. Might Hatfull have something in his catalogue of phages that could work against this patient's *M. abscessus*?

Hatfull and his team tested the girl's isolate against their collection and came up with a few potential matches – 'but not very many, and we had to look really hard to find them amongst our collection,' he says. There's another step to finding effective phages, however. For phages to kill bacteria, they need to be 'lytic', causing lysis of the cell by rupturing the cell membrane. But some phages, known as temperate phages, don't always do this. They may kill bacterial cells most of the time, but sometimes they are instead 'lysogenic', which means they enter the bacterial cell but then become incorporated within it, allowing the bacteria to survive. 'A phage that only kills 90 per cent of the time isn't going to be very good therapeutically, because 10 per cent of quite a lot of bacteria is still a lot of bacteria,' Hatfull says.

Not only do you need to find the right phages for a particular bacterial infection, then; they must also be lytic ones. But many phages in Hatfull and his team's collection are temperate – including two of the three they wanted to combine into a cocktail to treat this patient.

Their solution? Genome editing. They engineered the genomes of the phages such that they would always be lytic, by removing the genes needed for lysogeny. By doing this, Hatfull explains, 'We've essentially converted a naturally occurring temperate phage into one that's now lytic, and essentially moved it from the "can't use" category into the "potential use" category.' He credits the basic biology his lab has been doing for the fact that they had such tools at their disposal; only by studying the genetics of phages did they have the knowledge and ability to do this engineering.

To decide on the details of how to administer the phages, Hatfull and his colleagues worked with Chip Schooley, who had been instrumental in Patterson's treatment. Again, they had very little to go on; there is no real known optimal dose for intravenous phage therapy. They decided on a dose of a billion phage particles, twice a day. Giving such an experimental treatment, says Hatfull, is scary: 'You spend a lot of time thinking about all the things that could go wrong, and then worrying about all the things that [you're] not smart enough to think about.'

The treatment, as Hatfull and colleagues reported in *Nature Medicine*, was well tolerated, and the girl's condition improved.[17] It took a few weeks, but there was a reduction in bacterial load, the wound from her lung transplant closed, and her skin cleared up. Since this experience, Hatfull has been approached by many physicians – he estimates more than 200 – who are interested in exploring phage therapy for their patients. But at the moment, in the US at least, phage therapy is still very experimental, permitted only on a case-by-case basis when there is no alternative.

For his part, Hatfull says he remains sceptical about whether phages will ever become a common therapy. In their paper on the *M. abscessus* case, the researchers noted that the patient's condition might have improved anyway – it's hard to draw solid conclusions from a one-off attempt. Clinical trials will be needed to see if phages could have widespread application.

One particular challenge with using phages on a larger scale is their specificity – the fact that they need to be tailored to a particular bacterial isolate rather than just a species of bacteria. This, Hatfull says, is 'the critical factor that has complicated the advancement of phage therapy in the big picture'. Tailoring a treatment to an individual is expensive and time-consuming, and would make it difficult to adopt phage therapy as a straightforward alternative to antibiotics.

Perhaps, Hatfull suggests, phages could be a boutique treatment for certain infections where patients have little other recourse. Or they could be useful as an adjunct to antibiotics to treat specific infections, if clinical trials show that combining the two therapies leads to better results. A future approach to phage therapy could be to design and make them synthetically, engineering them to be maximally effective. This could potentially help with the problem of specificity: if you could engineer a phage so that it works against more bacterial strains, maybe it would be possible to deploy it more broadly.

All of this is a long way off – there are regulatory and commercial hurdles as well as scientific ones to overcome – but research groups and companies are starting to study phage therapy with renewed interest. Strathdee is now co-director of UCSD's Center for Innovative Phage Applications and Therapeutics, which she founded with Chip Schooley in 2018 and which treats patients with phages on a case-by-case basis according to the FDA's compassionate use programme.

She also sees phages as a potential adjunct to, rather than replacement for, antibiotics. In her husband's case, the bacteria mutated to stop the phages from working, but in doing so made themselves more vulnerable for one of the antibiotics to attack. 'So that kind of synergy where phages and antibiotics can be used together can be very powerful,' she says.

She hopes that phage therapy will allow us to use fewer antibiotics – crucial for keeping resistance at bay. As well as being used in medicine, perhaps they could find applications in veterinary care, agriculture or aquaculture. It's early days. But based on her experience, she is keen to act as an advocate for phage therapy.

She recognises that she and Patterson were incredibly privileged to have access to the resources they did. 'The majority of people dying from superbug infections are in low-resource settings that don't have access,' she says.

Conclusion: Not rocket science

Innovations in science and technology offer fertile ground for exploring different ways to tackle antimicrobial resistance. But ultimately, the things that could have the most impact are the ones we already know about – things like access to clean water and sanitation, infection prevention and control measures, and improved access to existing vaccines and treatments. 'The fact is, we shouldn't have people getting infected in the first place,' says Wellcome's Tim Jinks.

If we can help prevent people from getting ill to begin with – by making sure they have toilets and clean drinking water, for instance – then we will automatically reduce the spread of infection and the need for antimicrobials. Similarly, if we can improve infection control measures in hospitals, we will reduce the spread of hospital-acquired infections. This, Jinks says, is 'not going to require some mad genius to come up with the transformative thing. It's the willingness and dedication to implement known tools and practices to achieve that.'

When people do get infections, we need to be better at treating them – using the right antimicrobials in the right patients, at the right doses. We need to have better diagnostics to make sure we're using the correct drugs, and better surveillance to head off resistance threats before they snowball. We need to keep developing antimicrobials, and when we bring them to market we need to be even better at applying antimicrobial stewardship to hold off the emergence of resistance as long as possible. We also need to reconsider our use of antimicrobials in agriculture and the environment.

It's a constant battle fought on many fronts, but it's one that we all can help with. Individuals can refrain from asking for antibiotics when they have a cold and follow the instructions when they are prescribed them.

Prescribers can make sure they're sticking to stewardship guidelines. And policymakers can start thinking longer term about how to address an issue that isn't going away any time soon.

The scale of the problem requires a collaborative approach, says Jessica Boname, of the UK's Medical Research Council. A multitude of solutions are needed to address the many different issues related to antimicrobial resistance around the world. Just as we have seen with the Covid-19 pandemic, we need researchers, clinicians, engineers, politicians, behavioural scientists and economists to work together across borders. 'We won't succeed if we're only trying to fix things in our own backyard,' she says. 'We want to make sure that we provide a suite of solutions, which will support people living in different contexts and who have different problems.'

The issue of antimicrobial resistance may not seem urgent. It's not a tsunami, a forest fire, a sudden viral outbreak. But as long as we fail to stop infections spreading and continue to overuse antimicrobials without a thought to the long-term consequences, the threat will continue to build. More people will die. The best time to take action is now.

Acknowledgements

Thank you to all of those who took the time to share their knowledge and experience during my reporting of this book, particularly David Aanensen, Emily Adams, Hazel Barton, Daniel Berman, Silvia Bertagnolio, Jessica Boname, Naowarat Cheeptham, Jim Collins, Nicholas Croucher, Sachin Dubey, Slava Epstein, Nicholas Feasey, Matthew Fisher, Graham Hatfull, Kat Holt, Tim Jinks, Gwen Knight, Kim Lewis, Danilo Lo Fo Wong, Cal MacLennan, Greg McCallum, Matt Mulvey, Ruth Neale, Helen Osment, Kevin Outterson, Jan Poolman, Gary Schoolnik, Ayesha Sitlani, Steffanie Strathdee, Mat Upton, Dalene Von Delft, Mark Webber, Nicholas White, Gerry Wright and Muhammad Zaman.

The issue of antimicrobial resistance is a broad one, with many different facets. It would be impossible for this book to attempt to cover them all, but I hope it serves as a useful introduction to some of the key points. Books I would recommend as a starting point for those interested in learning more include: *The Drugs Don't Work: A Global Threat*, by Professor Dame Sally C. Davies; *Biography of Resistance: The Epic Battle Between People and Pathogens*, by Muhammad H. Zaman; *The Perfect Predator: A Scientist's Race to Save Her Husband From a Deadly Superbug*, by Steffanie Strathdee and Thomas Patterson. Maryn McKenna's writing on antimicrobial resistance, for WIRED and elsewhere, is always a good read.

Thank you most of all to all of the scientists, clinicians, policymakers, activists, advocates and others who are working to reduce the impact of antimicrobial resistance around the world. Your hard work and dedication is quite literally saving lives.

Finally, thank you to my editors at WIRED and Penguin. And thank you to Henry, for his enduring patience and support.

Notes

Notes to Introduction:

The post-antimicrobial world   pages 1–7

1   covid19.who.int, accessed 12 March 2022

2   https://www.thelancet.com/journals/lancet/article/
       PIIS0140-6736(21)02724-0/fulltext#%20

3   cdc.gov/drugresistance/biggest-threats.html

4   https://www.nhtsa.gov/press-releases/2020-fatality-data-
       show-increased-traffic-fatalities-during-pandemic

5   https://www.who.int/news-room/fact-sheets/detail/
       antibiotic-resistance

Notes to 1 Resistance rising   pages 12–37

1   https://www.bmj.com/content/358/bmj.j3402.full

2   https://amr-review.org/sites/default/files/160525_
       Final%20paper_with%20cover.pdf

3   https://www.britannica.com/biography/Alexander-Fleming

4   https://www.acs.org/content/acs/en/education/
    whatischemistry/landmarks/flemingpenicillin.html

5   https://www.nobelprize.org/uploads/2018/06/fleming-
    lecture.pdf

6   Ibid.

7   https://journals.plos.org/plosbiology/article?id=10.1371/
    journal.pbio.1002533

8   https://www.nice.org.uk/Media/Default/About/what-we-
    do/NICE-guidance/antimicrobial%20guidance/summary-
    antimicrobial-prescribing-guidance.pdf

9   https://royalsocietypublishing.org/doi/10.1098/
    rspb.2018.0789

10 http://www.aimspress.com/article/10.3934/
    microbiol.2018.3.482

11 https://www.nature.com/articles/nature10388

12 https://advances.sciencemag.org/content/1/3/e1500183

13 https://journals.plos.org/plosone/article?id=10.1371/
    journal.pone.0034953

14 https://www.nice.org.uk/news/article/antibiotic-
    resistance-is-now-common-in-urinary-tract-infections

15   https://www.nytimes.com/2019/07/13/health/urinary-infections-drug-resistant.html

16   Muhammad H. Zaman, *Biography of Resistance: The Epic Battle Between People and Pathogens,* HarperWave, 2020

17   A. Doble et al., 'Antibiotic prescribing and resistance: Views from low- and middle-income prescribing and dispensing professionals', 2018.

18   https://amr-review.org/sites/default/files/ElizabethPisaniMedicinesQualitypaper.pdf

19   https://www.thelancet.com/journals/lancet/article/PIIS0140-6736(19)32798-9/fulltext

20   Swann Committee, 'Report of Joint Committee on the Use of Antibiotics in Animal Husbandry and Veterinary Medicine', 1969

21   https://www.nature.com/articles/s41599-018-0152-2

22   https://muse.jhu.edu/article/698175

23   https://www.saveourantibiotics.org/media/1808/swann-song-for-routine-antibiotic-use.pdf

24   https://www.who.int/news/item/07-11-2017-stop-using-antibiotics-in-healthy-animals-to-prevent-the-spread-of-antibiotic-resistance

25 https://www.thelancet.com/journals/lancet/article/
PIIS0140-6736(19)32306-2/fulltext

26 https://www.thelancet.com/journals/lancet/article/
PIIS0140-6736(15)00474-2/fulltext

27 https://www.bloomberg.com/news/articles/2019-09-05/
superbugs-deadlier-than-cancer-put-chemotherapy-into-
question

Notes to 2 Meet the superbugs
1 https://www.clinicalmicrobiologyandinfection.com/
article/S1198-743X(14)61632-3/fulltext

2 https://www.who.int/news-room/fact-sheets/detail/the-
top-10-causes-of-death

3 https://apps.who.int/iris/bitstream/handle/
10665/336069/9789240013131-eng.pdf

4 https://cdn.who.int/media/docs/default-source/
hq-tuberculosis/who_globalhbcliststb_2021-2025_
backgrounddocument.pdf?sfvrsn=f6b854c2_9

5 https://www.who.int/news-room/fact-sheets/detail/
antimicrobial-resistance

6   https://www.who.int/news-room/q-a-detail/tuberculosis-
      multidrug-resistant-tuberculosis-(mdr-tb)

7   https://www.cdc.gov/hai/patientsafety/ar-hospitals.html

8   https://www.who.int/news/item/27-02-2017-who-
      publishes-list-of-bacteria-for-which-new-antibiotics-are-
      urgently-needed

9   https://asm.org/Protocols/Gram-Stain-Protocols

10   https://apps.who.int/iris/bitstream/handle/
      10665/330420/9789240000193-eng.pdf

11   https://www.cdc.gov/mmwr/volumes/66/wr/mm6601a7.
      htm?s_cid=mm6601a7_w

12   https://www.cancer.gov/publications/dictionaries/cancer-
      terms/def/systemic-inflammatory-response-syndrome

13   https://www.cdc.gov/drugresistance/biggest-threats.
      html#cdiff

14   https://www.ecdc.europa.eu/en/clostridium-difficile-
      infections/facts

15   https://www.cdc.gov/cdiff/what-is.html#again

16   https://www.thelancet.com/journals/laninf/article/
      PIIS1473-3099(20)30120-1/fulltext

17   https://www.thelancet.com/journals/lanres/article/
     PIIS2213-2600(21)00265-4/fulltext#%20

18   https://science.sciencemag.org/content/360/6390/739

19   https://aricjournal.biomedcentral.com/articles/10.1186/
     s13756-016-0132-5

20   https://www.nytimes.com/2019/04/06/health/drug-
     resistant-candida-auris.html

Notes to 3 The search for new antibiotics   pages 72–98

1   https://www.who.int/news/item/17-01-2020-lack-of-new-
     antibiotics-threatens-global-efforts-to-contain-drug-
     resistant-infections

2   https://journals.asm.org/doi/10.1128/CMR.00030-10

3   https://science.sciencemag.org/content/311/5759/374

4   https://www.nature.com/articles/nature10388

5   https://www.nature.com/articles/ncomms13803

6   https://www.nature.com/articles/nbt.2685

7   https://www.nature.com/articles/s41586-020-1990-9

8   https://www.nature.com/articles/nature14098

9   https://www.cell.com/cell/fulltext/S0092-8674(20)30102-1

10 https://www.who.int/news/item/27-02-2017-who-publishes-list-of-bacteria-for-which-new-antibiotics-are-urgently-needed

11 https://digitalcommons.law.yale.edu/yjhple/vol5/iss1/4/

12 https://www.gov.uk/government/news/world-first-scheme-underway-to-tackle-amr-and-protect-uk-patients

13 https://www.england.nhs.uk/blog/how-the-nhs-model-to-tackle-antimicrobial-resistance-amr-can-set-a-global-standard/

14 https://www.statnews.com/2021/06/25/pasteur-act-help-fight-superbugs-antimicrobial-resistance/

Notes to 4 Diagnostics and surveillance   pages 101–124

1 https://www.theguardian.com/science/2014/may/18/true-sea-shanty-story-behind-longitude-prize-john-harrison

2 https://www.who.int/news/item/08-09-2020-who-calls-for-global-action-on-sepsis---cause-of-1-in-5-deaths-worldwide

3 https://academic.oup.com/jid/article/183/Supplement_1/S1/2190986

4   https://www.nih.gov/news-events/news-releases/rapid-diagnostic-gonorrhea-wins-19-million-federal-prize-competition-combat-antibiotic-resistance

5   https://assets.publishing.service.gov.uk/government/uploads/system/uploads/attachment_data/file/701185/hpr1418_MDRGC.pdf

6   https://www.thelancet.com/pdfs/journals/laninf/PIIS1473-3099(20)30734-9.pdf

7   https://www.who.int/initiatives/glass/glass-routine-data-surveillance

8   https://www.who.int/publications/i/item/9789240027336

9   https://journals.plos.org/plosntds/article?id=10.1371/journal.pntd.0003748

10   https://www.nejm.org/doi/full/10.1056/NEJMoa2035916

11   https://www.who.int/publications/i/item/9789240027336

12   https://www.ecdc.europa.eu/sites/default/files/documents/shigella-infections-men-sex-men-february-2022-erratum.pdf

13   https://www.nature.com/articles/s41598-018-25764-3

14   https://www.gov.uk/government/news/rise-in-
     extremely-drug-resistant-shigella-in-gay-and-
     bisexual-men

Notes to 5 Antibiotic alternatives   pages 130–154

1   https://www.who.int/news-room/feature-stories/detail/
     how-do-vaccines-work

2   https://vk.ovg.ox.ac.uk/vk/types-of-vaccine

3   https://www.gatesfoundation.org/our-work/programs/
     global-health/enteric-and-diarrheal-diseases

4   https://apps.who.int/iris/bitstream/handle/
     10665/277258/9789241565691-eng.pdf

5   https://www.birmingham.ac.uk/research/immunology-
     immunotherapy/research/bactivac/funded-projects/prof-
     calman-maclennan.aspx

6   https://www.euro.who.int/en/health-topics/
     diseaseprevention/antimicrobial-resistance/news/
     news/2015/10/vaccinating-salmon-how-norway-avoids-
     antibiotics-infish-farming

7 https://www.newscientist.com/definition/antibodies/

8 https://www.iavi.org/news-resources/expanding-access-to-monoclonal-antibody-based-products-a-global-call-to-action

9 Ibid.

10 https://www.legion.org/magazine/1516/iraqibacter

11 https://www.ncbi.nlm.nih.gov/pmc/articles/PMC5346588/

12 https://www.nature.com/scitable/definition/bacteriophage-phage-293/

13 https://www.tandfonline.com/doi/full/10.4161/bact.1.1.14942

14 https://www.cell.com/trends/microbiology/fulltext/S0966-842X(12)00225-9

15 Steffanie Strathdee and Thomas Patterson, *The Perfect Predator: A Scientist's Race to Save Her Husband from a Deadly Superbug* (Hachette, 2019)

16 https://www.sciencemag.org/news/2019/05/viruses-genetically-engineered-kill-bacteria-rescue-girl-antibiotic-resistant-infection

17 https://www.nature.com/articles/s41591-019-0437-z

Index